# O A P L
OXFORD AMERICAN PSYCHIATRY LIBRARY

## Schizophrenia

D1166852

# O A P L
## OXFORD AMERICAN PSYCHIATRY LIBRARY

# Schizophrenia

## Stephen R. Marder, MD

Professor of Psychiatry and Biobehavioral Sciences
David Geffen School of Medicine at UCLA
Los Angeles, CA

**Associate Author: Vandana Chopra, MD**

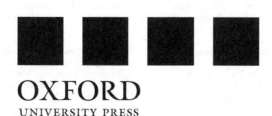

OXFORD
UNIVERSITY PRESS

# OXFORD
UNIVERSITY PRESS

Oxford University Press is a department of the University of
Oxford. It furthers the University's objective of excellence in research,
scholarship, and education by publishing worldwide.

Oxford   New York
Auckland   Cape Town   Dar es Salaam   Hong Kong   Karachi
Kuala Lumpur   Madrid   Melbourne   Mexico City   Nairobi
New Delhi   Shanghai   Taipei   Toronto

With offices in
Argentina   Austria   Brazil   Chile   Czech Republic   France   Greece
Guatemala   Hungary   Italy   Japan   Poland   Portugal   Singapore
South Korea   Switzerland   Thailand   Turkey   Ukraine   Vietnam

Oxford is a registered trademark of Oxford University Press
in the UK and certain other countries.

Published in the United States of America by
Oxford University Press
198 Madison Avenue, New York, NY 10016

© Oxford University Press 2014

Library of Congress Cataloging-in-Publication Data
Marder, Stephen R., 1945- author
Schizophrenia / Stephen R. Marder ; associate author, Vandana Chopra.
   p. ; cm.—(Oxford American psychiatry library)
Includes bibliographical references.
ISBN 978-0-19-996465-9 (alk. paper)
I. Chopra, Vandana, author.   II. Title.   III. Series: Oxford American psychiatry library.
[DNLM: 1. Schizophrenia. WM 203]
RC514
616.89′8—dc23          2014019489

This material is not intended to be, and should not be considered, a substitute for medical
or other professional advice. Treatment for the conditions described in this material is highly
dependent on the individual circumstances. And, while this material is designed to offer
accurate information with respect to the subject matter covered and to be current as of the
time it was written, research and knowledge about medical and health issues is constantly
evolving and dose schedules for medications are being revised continually, with new side
effects recognized and accounted for regularly. Readers must therefore always check the
product information and clinical procedures with the most up-to-date published product
information and data sheets provided by the manufacturers and the most recent codes
of conduct and safety regulation. The publisher and the authors make no representations
or warranties to readers, express or implied, as to the accuracy or completeness of
this material. Without limiting the foregoing, the publisher and the authors make no
representations or warranties as to the accuracy or efficacy of the drug dosages mentioned
in the material. The authors and the publisher do not accept, and expressly disclaim, any
responsibility for any liability, loss or risk that may be claimed or incurred as a consequence
of the use and/or application of any of the contents of this material.

9 8 7 6 5 4 3 2 1
Printed in the United States of America
on acid-free paper

# Contents

# Contents

Dr. Marder has served as a paid consultant for the following companies: Abbvie, EnVivo, Targacept, Roche, Pfizer, Lundbeck, Boeringer-Ingelheim, Otsuka. He has received grant support from Amgen, Sunovion, Genentech, and Psychogenics.

Dr. Vandana Chopra has no known conflicts to disclose.

# O A P L

OXFORD AMERICAN PSYCHIATRY LIBRARY

# Schizophrenia

# Chapter 1

# Introduction

There is no such thing as a typical person with schizophrenia. Individuals can vary from those who are tormented by unremitting refractory psychotic symptoms to those who have a relatively minor symptom burden, from those who are recovering from a recent psychotic episode to those who live in their communities burdened by chronic impairments and medication side effects, and from those who are in the midst of their first episode to those who have lived with their illnesses for decades. The processes for managing these diverse groups of patients require an ability to adapt the evaluation process and to tailor the interventions to an individual's needs.

This volume has adapted to this reality by organizing its sections around different patient groups and different stages of the disorder. Each of these sections includes recommendations for evaluating patients and for management strategies that are appropriate for particular clinical situations. Since treatment often requires integrating pharmacological and psychosocial treatments, both are included with each section. We anticipate that this approach will emphasize the importance of designing treatments based on an individual's disease burden as well as his or her personal goals.

We have also incorporated principles of recovery into patient management. This includes emphasizing patient-centered care that is driven by an individual's personal goals and priorities. Management recommendations emphasize a strategy that helps patients to meet their goals even if symptoms and impairments persist. We have also tried to convey appropriate optimism regarding the ability of many patients to meet their own goals for recovery.

Nearly all of the recommendations in this text are supported by a firm evidence base. In many cases we have cited authoritative evidence reviews such as the Schizophrenia PORT (Schizophrenia Patient Outcomes Research Team) (1). Where there is inadequate evidence to support a recommendation, we have also cited expert opinions, including our own. Our overall intention is to assist clinicians as they address the complex and challenging issues that they face in treating individuals who present to them with clinical problems that include symptoms of schizophrenia.

## References

1. Kreyenbuhl J, Buchanan RW, Dickerson FB, Dixon LB, Schizophrenia Patient Outcomes Research Team. The Schizophrenia Patient Outcomes Research Team (PORT): updated treatment recommendations 2009. *Schizophr Bull.* 2010;36(1):94–103.

# Chapter 2

# Evaluation and Management of Acute Psychosis

## Evaluation of the Acutely Psychotic Patient

Patients with psychotic symptoms are first seen in a variety of clinical settings, including the offices of primary care providers, psychiatrists, non-physician mental healthcare providers (psychologists, social workers, nurses, and others), and emergency rooms.

Essential issues to be considered in the initial evaluation include the following:

1. The safety of the patient and those who interact with the patient;
2. Personal discomfort the patient may be experiencing from psychotic experiences;
3. Assuring that the psychosis is not related to a medical condition that requires immediate treatment;
4. Assessing the ability of the patient to participate in decisions about his or her management;
5. Deciding about the best place for the patient to receive treatment.

Considering medical causes of an acute psychosis should occur very early in the evaluation. Causes may include alcohol or drug use, neurological or endocrine disorders, sepsis, and cardiovascular disorders. Obtaining vital signs, determining that the patient is oriented, performing a neurological examination, and ruling out causes such as hypoxia or hypoglycemia should be part of evaluating any new psychosis.

Some clinicians may be uncomfortable with making management decisions and beginning treatment before reaching a diagnosis. However, obtaining an adequate history from the patient, family members, and other providers may be impossible during the initial evaluation, when psychotic symptoms may be most acute. Also, the initial treatments for any psychosis are not disease specific. That is, pharmacological and psychosocial approaches to acute psychosis are similar whether the underlying disorder is schizophrenia, a psychotic mood disorder, or an organic psychosis.

## Evaluation for Safety in the Emergency Room

There are a number of factors to consider in assessing the risk of violent or self-destructive behavior in individuals with schizophrenia and other psychotic illnesses (1–3).

The following factors are associated with a risk of violent behavior in psychotic individuals:

• A history of violent behavior
• Concerns of individuals close to the patient regarding threats
• Command hallucinations
• Comorbid substance use
• History of impulsive behavior
• Male gender are at a greater risk for violence.

The following factors are associated with a risk for self-destructive and suicidal behaviors:

• A history of suicidal behavior
• Command hallucinations
• Comorbid substance use
• Young age.

In the emergency room, organic contributors to aggressive behavior should be ruled out, even if the patient is known to have a history of a psychotic illness. Drug and alcohol intoxication are probably the most common causes of violence in the emergency room (4). Other common causes are post-ictal states, hypoglycemia, and withdrawal syndromes, particularly with alcohol. Patients who appear angry or aggressive should be interviewed in a room where both the patient and the clinician have access to a door. Verbal approaches to calming the patient should be used whenever possible. These include approaching the patient in a friendly and supportive manner and showing an interest in the patient's concerns. Physical restraints should only be used when other approaches are unsuccessful.

The results of the safety assessment will determine how urgently the clinician needs to make decisions to protect the safety of the patient and others. It is important for the clinician to address these safety considerations directly by asking patients about their current psychotic experiences and whether they involve people in their immediate environment. Hallucinations commanding the patient to carry out violent acts against themselves or others should alert the clinician that there is a safety issue—even if the patient appears relatively calm (5). These experiences are particularly dangerous when the patient reports that it is difficult to resist the commands. Delusional ideas about people in the patient's environment should also raise concerns if the patient believes that he or she has no choice but to act.

Family members and other informants may also provide valuable information about the patient's recent behavior and their thought content. This may be particularly helpful when it is difficult or impossible to obtain an adequate history from the patient.

## History and Physical Evaluation

### History of Present Illness

As with any psychiatric interview, the patient should be approached with an open-ended "How can I help you today?" and then be permitted to answer in an uninterrupted fashion for at least 3–5 minutes. During this time, the patient will often reveal his chief complaint and any other primary psychotic symptoms, allowing the clinician to tailor the remainder of the interview accordingly. Whenever possible, direct quotes from the patient documenting the reason for current presentation should be recorded.

Some patients with active psychotic symptoms or negative symptoms may provide little or no information when they are asked open-ended questions. If this is the case, the clinician should ask for any remaining information directly. Asking, "Why did you come to see me today instead of yesterday or last week?" can often provide clues to what the main target symptoms are and how these have grown unbearable or how functioning has been negatively impacted. It is important to understand in what ways baseline functioning has been altered. Asking for a detailed description of how the patient spent the waking hours of his day prior to presentation can provide this useful information.

Eliciting reports of psychotic symptoms can be challenging when patients are guarded or suspicious. Inquiring if the person has felt that she is in danger or if there are particular people or circumstances that she is avoiding may lead to useful descriptions of reality distortions. Individuals with psychotic experiences may find it difficult to be in places that are noisy or overstimulating. Asking if the patient has strange or unusual thoughts may also elicit descriptions of psychotic symptoms.

A description of any other symptoms related to the current episode should also be gathered, including any hallucinations (command or otherwise), delusions, paranoia, changes in mood (depression or mania), anxiety or cognition, changes in speech or behavior, and/or social isolation. Documenting the noted absence of these symptoms can be useful, especially to clinicians who may be evaluating the patient at a future point in time.

Understanding recent events in the patient's life may provide information about potential triggers to the patient's psychotic episode. Have there been any particular changes to the patient's environment recently? Were there any noted or reported physical changes that accompanied or preceded this episode (increased pain, somatic complaints, weight loss, etc.)? Other possible triggers may be any new or increased drug use (illicit or prescribed). Finally, the clinician may also consider possible motives for secondary gain, especially if the patient's history is somewhat inconsistently presented. A few common reasons that patients might feign or exaggerate psychotic symptoms are to secure disability payments (perhaps in concert with an untreated substance abuse problem) or to secure housing in the context of current homelessness.

## Past Psychiatric History

A list of previous psychiatric diagnoses, age of illness onset as well as type, and duration and effectiveness of any intervention (medications, hospitalizations, or day treatment programs, social skills or vocational therapy, family therapy, etc.) should be recorded here. Whether the patient's illness has been steadily improving or worsening can also impact clinical decision-making and therefore is an important determination to make. The history should also include descriptions of the earliest signs that the person was becoming psychotic.

Contacting current and previous providers (with the patient's permission) can provide valuable information related to verifying information obtained in the history of present illness (HPI). Previous clinicians may also describe any particular barriers to treatment, any recent challenges faced by the patient, and whether there are any comorbid psychiatric illnesses (for example, ongoing substance abuse or difficult personality traits) that may further impact current treatment. From the patient's perspective, learning what aspects of therapy or what characteristics of the therapist were most helpful may be useful when attempting to quickly establish a new therapeutic alliance.

The circumstances regarding any previous hospitalizations should also be documented; the number of hospitalizations, date of last discharge, average length of stay, and whether admission was voluntary or involuntary can provide a fuller understanding of the patient's overall clinical trajectory to date.

Finally, it is important to note whether the patient has a history of self-injurious behaviors or a history of suicidal ideation, threats, or attempts. Similarly, any assaultive behaviors or violence toward others and the circumstances surrounding these episodes should also be carefully documented.

## Medication History

The medication history should minimally include the names, dosages, duration, outcome, and side effects, as well as time of last administration. Clinicians should ask patients specifically about any neurological symptoms, including restlessness and stiffness as well as weight gain. Obtaining additional useful information, such as a patient's prior non-adherence with treatment and whether the patient required medication management by others, can be extremely helpful for creating a treatment plan.

## Medical History

A current list of medical problems, including ongoing uncontrolled symptoms, should be carefully recorded and continually updated. Documenting any history of head trauma, seizures, brain tumors, or any previous surgeries is highly relevant. A detailed tobacco history should also be taken.

For patients with an acute psychosis, a number of medical conditions that can cause or worsen psychosis should be considered. These are summarized in Table 2.1.

## Assessment Before Drug Treatment

Whenever possible, patients should have a physical examination and laboratory tests prior to starting an antipsychotic. Since acute treatment with antipsychotics is relatively safe, there are circumstances—particularly when patients are agitated or aggressive—when medications can be started without the preferred evaluation. However, attempts should be made to assure that patients have their vital signs assessed whenever possible.

## Table 2.1 Medical Conditions Known to Cause Acute Psychosis

| Medical Condition | Description |
| --- | --- |
| **Neurologic** | |
| Narcolepsy | Excessive daytime sleepiness, cataplexy, sleep paralysis, and hypnagogic hallucinations |
| Seizure | Particularly temporal lobe epilepsy. Can occur during all ictal phases. |
| Space occupying lesion | Brain tumors, particularly temporal lobe location. Focal midbrain lesions can cause peduncular hallucinosis. Conditions that increase intracranial pressure (for example, normal pressure hydrocephalus). |
| Stroke | Most commonly, stroke-related seizure activity is responsible. Charles Bonnet syndrome (visual hallucinations) following occipital infarction. |
| Demyelinating disease | Disruption of white matter tracts can lead to psychosis, likely due to functional disconnection of critical brain regions. |
| Inherited leukodystrophies (metachromatic leukodystrophy [MLD] or adrenoleukodystrophy [ALD]) | High prevalence of neuropsychiatric symptoms, including psychosis, progressive cognitive decline, seizures |
| Basal ganglia disorders (rare: Wilson, Huntington, Fahr; and more common: Parkinson's disease) | Psychosis including hallucinations, most commonly visual with Parkinson's disease |
| **Endocrine** | |
| Thyroid | Hyperthyroidism, hypothyroidism (myxedema madness), Hashimoto encephalopathy |
| Steroid-producing tumor | Adrenal (Cushing disease), small cell lung cancer (ectopic Cushing disease) |
| Insulinoma | Confusion, bizarre behavior |
| Pheochromocytoma | |
| **Nutritional** | |
| Nutritional deficiencies | Psychosis from vitamin B12 deficiency, thiamine deficiency |
| **Mechanical** | |
| Traumatic brain injury | Usually paranoid-hallucinatory syndrome that can continue to develop several years after injury |
| Toxins | Carbon monoxide; organophosphates; and heavy metals, particularly arsenic, manganese, mercury, and thallium |
| Metabolic | Acute intermittent porphyria (AIP), Tay-Sachs disease, Niemann-Pick disease type C (rare) |

*(Continued)*

**Table 2.1 (Continued)**

| Medical Condition | Description |
|---|---|
| Autoimmune | Systemic lupus erythematosus (SLE), paraneoplastic limbic encephalitis (PLE) |
| **Infectious** | |
| Including immigrant populations or travelers | Including cerebral malaria, toxoplasmosis, neurocysticercosis, herpes simplex encephalitis; also HIV infection and neurosyphilis |

### Assessment Prior to Starting an Antipsychotic

- Vital signs (heart rate, blood pressure)
- Body mass index (BMI)
- Waist circumference
- Signs of a movement disorder:
    - Extrapyramidal symptoms (EPS): akathisia, Parkinsonism, dystonias
    - Tardive dyskinesia: abnormal movements of the face, peri-oral areas, tongue, extremities.

Laboratory tests (with the exception of a neutrophil count for patients receiving clozapine, the antipsychotic can usually be started before the results of laboratory tests are available):

- CBC, electrolytes, fasting glucose, lipid profile, liver, renal and thyroid function tests
- ECG for patients with a cardiac history or those being treated with anti-psychotics that may prolong the QT interval such as clozapine, thioridazine, iloperidone, ziprasidone.

## Management of Agitation

When patients with psychosis are agitated, there is a tendency to start a medication right away. However, many patients can be calmed with non-pharmacological interventions. These can include supportive interactions with staff that help the suspicious patient feel safe or finding a quiet place for patients who are overly responsive to their environment. Approaching the patient in a reassuring and non-threatening manner can be calming for many individuals. It may also be helpful to maintain a distance between the provider and patient that seems greater than the distance for normal conversation. Allowing the patient to describe the thoughts and feelings that are the source of agitation can also be helpful. Challenging the patient's logic is seldom helpful when patients are agitated. Offering the patient something to eat or drink can also contribute to creating a calming environment.

Physical restraints should only be used as a last resort for the highly dangerous patient. The UK National Institute for Clinical Excellence (NICE) (http://publications.nice.org.uk/violence-cg25/guidance) specifies that physical restraint should only be used when there is a real possibility of significant harm if restraint is not used. Moreover, the minimal amount of restraint should always be used, and restraints should be removed as soon as possible. In some individuals, the restraints may actually increase the individual's level of agitation. In addition, under some conditions, restraints can be dangerous and they can elevate mortality rates. Restraints should be avoided whenever possible in patients with medical conditions.

Seclusion should also be used only when other interventions fail and when it is necessary for the safety of the patient and others. If the management goal is to calm the patient, a place should be used that is relatively quiet and where the individual can feel safe. In addition, seclusion should not be used as a punishment for bad behavior.

### Pharmacotherapy for Agitation

Either benzodiazepines or antipsychotics can be helpful for treating agitation in acutely psychotic patients. (Although benzodiazepines such as lorazepam are FDA approved for anxiety, they are commonly prescribed for patients with agitation.) If there is a concern that agitation is related to organic causes or substance use, benzodiazepines are preferred. In most other cases, an antipsychotic is preferred for patients who are both agitated and psychotic. Patients who are treated with an intramuscular (IM) antipsychotic will usually achieve an effective plasma concentration in less than 30 minutes. Although this can be an advantage in some circumstances, receiving an injection can contribute to agitation in some individuals who are mistrustful of the treatment team. As noted in Table 2.2, the maximum plasma concentration for an IM can come substantially sooner than with an oral agent, and patients may begin to experience the calming effects of an oral compound before reaching the maximum level. As a result, experienced clinicians are more likely to select an oral medication in patients who are willing to cooperate. Although oral solutions and oral disintegrating tablets may not reach effective levels before tablets, they can increase the confidence that the patient has swallowed the medication.

Although sedating antipsychotics such as quetiapine may be preferred by some patients and clinicians, minimally sedating antipsychotics have the advantage of providing a calming effect without sedation. If agitation is treated with repeated doses of an antipsychotic, there is a possibility that adverse effects, including hypotension, parkinsonism, akathisia, and sedation, will complicate management. For example, oral and parenteral antipsychotics may cause akathisia, an extrapyramidal side effect that can cause an experience of restlessness that increases agitation. Although akathisia is most commonly seen with high-potency antipsychotics such as haloperidol, aripiprazole, or ziprasidone, it can occur with any antipsychotic.

If patients remain agitated after one or two doses of an antipsychotic, it may be preferable to add a benzodiazepine such as lorazepam to induce calming.

## Inpatient or Outpatient Treatment

The decision regarding the setting for treatment depends largely on safety considerations, such as aggressive or self-injuring behaviors, or legal considerations for patients who are being treated involuntarily. Also, patients who are unable to follow instructions, those who require frequent monitoring, and patients who

## Table 2.2 Pharmacotherapy for Agitation

| | | Initial Dose (mg) | Max Dose for 24 hr | Time to Peak Plasma Conc (hrs) | |
|---|---|---|---|---|---|
| **Antipsychotics** | | | | | |
| Haloperidol | IM or IV | 2–5 | 30 | 0.5–1 | Severe risk of akathisia and dystonia |
| | Oral sol | 0.5–5 | 30 | 2 | |
| Fluphenazine | IM | 1.25 | 10 | 0.5 | Severe risk of akathisia and dystonia |
| | Oral sol | 1–2.5 | 10 | 3 | |
| Chlorpromazine | IM, IV | 25 | 200 | 0.5 | Severe risk of hypotension and sedation |
| Aripiprazole | IM | 9.75 | 20 | 1 | Observe for restlessness |
| | Oral sol and oral disintegrating tab | 10–15 | 20 | 3.5 | |
| Olanzapine | IM | 5–10 | 30 | 0.25–75 | |
| | Oral disintegrating tab | 5–10 | 20 | 5 | |
| Risperidone | Oral sol and oral disintegrating tab | 1–2 | 4 | 1.5 | |
| Ziprasidone | IM | 10–20 | 40 | 0.5–1 | Dose-related QTc prolongation |
| **Benzodiazepines** | | | | | |
| Lorazepam | IM or IV | 0.5–2 | 10 | 20–30 min | |
| | Oral | 0.5–4 | 10 | 2 hr | |
| Midazolam | IM | 2.5–5 | 10 | 0.5–1.0 hr | |
| | Oral sol | 1–2.5 | 10 | 3 | |
| Clonazepam | Oral | 1–3 | 20 | 1–3 hr | |

lack an adequate residence may require an inpatient admission. On the other hand, nearly any treatment for schizophrenia psychosis can be administered in an outpatient setting. There are advantages to being treated as an outpatient. Many patients will be more comfortable in the familiar surroundings of their own home. In addition, psychiatry wards can be overstimulating at a time when an acutely psychotic individual may benefit from an environment that is relatively peaceful.

## Pharmacological Treatment of Acute Psychosis

### Selecting an Antipsychotic

Nearly every acute psychosis should be treated with an antipsychotic medication. The selection of an antipsychotic should be based on a number of

## Table 2.3 Adverse Effects of Commonly Prescribed Antipsychotic Medications

| Antipsychotics | Extra-pyramidal Effects | Hypo-tension | Sedation | Weight Gain, Insulin Resistance, Lipid Elevation | Anti-cholin-ergic Effects |
|---|---|---|---|---|---|
| Haloperidol | +++ | + | + | + | + |
| Chlorpromazine | ++ | +++ | +++ | +++ | +++ |
| Fluphenazine | +++ | + | + | + | + |
| Perphenazine | ++ | + | ++ | + | + |
| Risperidone | ++ | ++ | + | ++ | + |
| Olanzapine | + | + | ++ | +++ | ++ |
| Clozapine | + | +++ | +++ | +++ | +++ |
| Quetiapine | + | ++ | +++ | ++ | + |
| Ziprasidone | + | + | + | + | + |
| Aripiprazole | + | + | + | + | + |
| Paliperidone | ++ | ++ | + | ++ | + |
| Iloperidone | + | +++ | + | ++ | + |
| Lurasidone | + | + | ++ | + | + |
| Asenapine | + | + | ++ | + | + |

+ none–mild, ++ moderate, +++ severe

considerations: prior history of response, patient's preference, available for-mulations, side effects, and cost. Table 2.3 lists a number of commonly pre-scribed antipsychotics, along with information about their side effects and dosing. Clozapine should be reserved for patients who have had relatively poor responses to at least two antipsychotics. Olanzapine should not be a first choice for younger patients since this group tends to be particularly sensitive to its metabolic effects (6). Low-potency first-generation antipsychotics such as chlorpromazine and thioridazine have side effect profiles that make them relatively undesirable for treating acute psychosis. That is, sedation and ortho-static hypotension occur commonly and require a gradual upward titration. In addition, high-potency first-generation agents such as haloperidol and fluphen-azine often cause extrapyramidal symptoms (EPS) at their therapeutic doses.

A number of large studies and meta-analyses have compared the effective-ness of different antipsychotics. Although some of these studies suggested that olanzapine and risperidone may be more effective than others, the dif-ferences were small and inconsistent among trials (7). The differences in side effects were substantial, with some antipsychotics causing substantial extrapy-ramidal side effects (including haloperidol and fluphenazine) and others (for example, clozapine and olanzapine) causing weight gain and other metabolic effects. Studies have shown that younger patients are particularly vulnerable to gaining weight on olanzapine (6). Other antipsychotics such as iloperidone and quetiapine require several days to reach a therapeutic level. As a result, these agents can add days to an inpatient stay.

Since there is no indication that there are differences in the efficacy of the available antipsychotics (with the exception of clozapine (8), which is more effective in patients who are partial responders on other antipsychotics), the selection of an antipsychotic will usually be made based on the side effects that the clinician wishes to avoid.

Patients who are acutely psychotic have often had unpleasant experiences with past antipsychotic drug trials. Since these patients may be drug reluctant, it is often helpful to have the patient play a significant role in deciding which antipsychotic will be started. For this process to be effective, the treating clinician should describe the side effects and possible benefits of each agent. Issues such as the availability of alternative formulations, the need for titration, and the possibility of once daily versus multiple daily dosing should be included in the conversation.

## Starting an Antipsychotic

Patients who are started on an antipsychotic will usually experience a side effect of the medication before they experience its therapeutic effects. The experience of an early side effect may lead a patient to conclude that he or she is unable to tolerate the drug, or that the medication's side effects are not balanced by therapeutic effects. A premature discontinuation of a medication can often be avoided by describing the side effects before administering the first dose. This can help assure that these early effects are described to the treatment team. Moreover, the description can support a collaborative and trusting relationship for patients who may tend to be suspicious.

If records are available, a past history of a drug response is probably the best source of information regarding drug dose. Otherwise, most patients should be started on a low to moderate therapeutic dose. Although there is an understandable inclination to treat more severely ill patients with higher doses of an antipsychotic, there is no indication that higher doses are more effective. Rather, antipsychotics appear to be effective when they reach doses that occupy 70% or more of $D_2$ dopamine receptors. Higher doses tend to contribute to a higher likelihood of side effects, but not to increased efficacy. In addition, there is no indication that higher doses are related to a more rapid response. Some antipsychotics such as olanzapine have relatively mild acute side effects, leading many psychiatrists to start patients on relatively high doses such as 30 mg daily or higher. The disadvantage of this high-dose strategy is that the clinician is unable to determine if the patient would have responded to a much lower dose. As a result, patients may remain on the higher dose after they have improved, exposing them to greater side effects.

In most patients, the response to an antipsychotic is delayed for several days. As a result, the clinician is unable to titrate the dose by assessing the drug's effectiveness. On the other hand, the side effects related to a drug dose can be assessed rather quickly. A reasonable dosing strategy is to start the patient on a low to moderate dose and assess how well the dose is tolerated. Adjustments to the starting dose can be made based on side effects. Patients will usually demonstrate whether they are responders to the initial regimen during the first 2 weeks of treatment. If patients fail to demonstrate any improvement during this period, the clinician should re-evaluate the treatment, possibly changing the dose or the antipsychotic. Most patients will not achieve a full remission of symptoms during this period. Rather, the existing symptoms may become less disturbing. For example, patients may describe auditory hallucinations as becoming softer, more friendly, or less frequent. Frightening delusions may become less frightening and the patient may be less distracted by delusions. Patients who misinterpreted the intentions of others may still have beliefs based on their prior misinterpretations. However, as they improve they may make fewer new misinterpretations. If patients are showing improvements such as these, they should be continued on the antipsychotic at the dose that is well tolerated. Most patients will continue to improve during subsequent weeks. Although individuals improve at different rates, an individual's responsiveness to an antipsychotic can usually be assessed after 6 weeks of treatment.

During the first days of inpatient treatment, prescribers may experience pressure from nursing staff and others to escalate the antipsychotic dose based on the belief that this will lead to a more rapid response. This can be a very understandable temptation, particularly when patients are receiving antipsychotics such as olanzapine that have relatively mild—and often pleasant—subjective side effects. However, most clinical studies have not shown that higher doses lead to more rapid responses when compared with the usual clinically recommended doses. Also, once patients are treated with a higher dose, it is unusual for clinicians to lower doses when patients have improved. The likely result is that the patient will continue to receive a higher dose than he or she actually requires.

After a trial of an antipsychotic for 6 weeks or more, patients may continue to have psychotic symptoms that are a minor annoyance and that do not affect their overall quality of life and community functioning. For these individuals, the antipsychotic should probably be continued at the current dose (unless there are side effects, as noted later on in this chapter). If, however, a patient continues to be disturbed by persisting psychotic symptoms, the plan should probably be reassessed. Strategies for managing persistent symptoms, including raising the dose, adding other agents, changing antipsychotics, adding clozapine, and cognitive behavioral therapy (CBT) for psychosis, are discussed in Chapter 6.

## Assessing and Managing Medication Side Effects

There are several side effects that are common during acute treatment. Side effects related to long-term treatment are discussed in Chapter 4. See Table 2.3 for side effects of commonly prescribed antipsychotics.

### Acute Extrapyramidal Side Effects

Although acute extrapyramidal side effects (EPS) are most common for high-potency antipsychotics—particularly high-potency first-generation antipsychotics such as haloperidol and fluphenazine—they can occur with any antipsychotic.

*Akathisia* is the most common form of acute EPS. It is relatively easy to recognize when patients are unable to sit or stand still. It can be difficult to recognize when patients are not moving but they are experiencing an inner sense of restlessness. Individuals with this subjective experience of restlessness can become agitated. This association of akathisia with agitation often leads to a difficult dilemma: Is a patient's increased agitation a result of too high an antipsychotic dose or inadequately treated psychosis? This problem is compounded when the patient is unable to describe his or her subjective experiences. One investigator (9) found that the most useful question for assessing akathisia was asking the patient whether it was difficult to sit still.

*Drug-induced Parkinsonism* is characterized by any of the symptoms of Parkinson's syndrome, including a mask-like facies, resting tremor, cogwheel rigidity, shuffling gait, and psychomotor retardation. Milder forms can appear as a lack of expressive gestures and facial expressions that appear apathetic. As a result, patients can appear to have negative symptoms of schizophrenia. If a clinician is uncertain whether a patient is having drug-induced Parkinsonism, it can be helpful to observe the patient walking. A decreased arm swing suggests Parkinsonism.

*Dystonias* are the most dramatic and the most disturbing EPS symptoms. Patients show involuntary contractions of muscle groups, often in the neck, jaw, and arms. Other patients may experience contractions of their eye muscles. On rare occasions, dystonias can affect the larynx and compromise respiration. Dystonias tend to occur early in antipsychotic treatment and are associated with high-potency first-generation antipsychotics such as haloperidol, particularly when administered intramuscularly.

### Treatment of Acute EPS

Acute EPS can often be managed by changing patients to an antipsychotic with a lower EPS liability or reducing the dose of the current antipsychotic.

Anticholinergic antiparkinson medications are effective for treating all forms of acute EPS. Patients can be started on an agent such as benztropine and prescribed 0.5 to 2 mg twice daily. These medications can have side effects related to their anticholinergic activity, including dry mouth, constipation, blurry vision, difficulty urinating in men, and memory impairment.

Akathisias can often be managed with dosage reduction. If this is ineffective, adding a beta blocker such as propranolol can be effective. Propranolol is usually started at 10 mg twice daily and can be increased to as much as 120 mg daily divided into 2 or 3 doses. The patient's blood pressure and heart rate should be monitored. Propranolol is contraindicated in patients with asthma or chronic obstructive pulmonary disease (COPD). It should not be discontinued abruptly since this can lead to tachycardia, hypertension, and ischemia. Akathisia can also be treated with benzodiazepines.

When dystonias are disturbing to patients they can be treated intramuscularly (IM) or even intravenously (IV) with 1 to 2 mg of benztropine or 50 mg of diphenhydramine. Since the onset of action is similar with IM or IV administration, IM is usually preferred. Milder dystonias can be treated with 1 or 2 mg of oral benztropine. Since dystonias can be severe reactions, their occurrence should lead to a re-evaluation of the patient's drug or a substantial lowering of the dose.

## Neuroleptic Malignant Syndrome

The neuroleptic malignant syndrome (NMS) is a serious, often life-threatening adverse reaction to antipsychotics that includes (1) fever, often greater than 104 degrees Fahrenheit; (2) severe muscle rigidity; (3) altered consciousness; and autonomic changes characterized by symptoms such as fluctuating blood pressure, tachypnea, and diaphoresis. The most common progression is that the mental status changes come first, followed by rigidity, fever, and then autonomic changes. Most patients with NMS have elevations in creatine kinase (CK). In many cases, CK levels can exceed 1000 IU/L and be as high as 100,000 IU/L. Diagnostic criteria proposed by an expert panel (10) are as follows:

- Recent dopamine antagonist exposure, or dopamine agonist withdrawal
- Hyperthermia (>100.4 degrees F or >38.0 degrees C on at least 2 occasions)
- Rigidity
- Mental status alteration, creatine kinase elevation (at least 4 times the upper limit of normal)
- Sympathetic nervous system lability (blood pressure elevation, ≥25% above baseline; blood pressure fluctuation, ≥20 mm Hg (diastolic) or ≥25 mm Hg (systolic) change within 24 hours)
- Tachycardia plus tachypnea (tachycardia, ≥25% above baseline; and tachypnea, ≥50% above baseline)
- A negative workup for other causes.

NMS can occur with any dopamine antagonist. It is most common when patients receive relatively high doses of first-generations antipsychotics and when doses are elevated rapidly. There are reports of NMS with second generation antipsychotics, including clozapine, although these are commonly associated with less rigidity and lower mortality (11). Most—but not all—cases of NMS occur during the first days of antipsychotic treatment.

NMS should be considered a medical emergency, and patients should be transferred to a medical setting. Progression of this syndrome can be rapid and can lead to rhabdomyolysis and multisystem organ failure. Dopamine antagonist treatments should be discontinued immediately. Medical care should be supportive and include managing unstable blood pressure, lowering the body temperature with cooling blankets and other measures when fever is high, managing tachycardia and tachypnea, and managing agitation with benzodiazepines. Since NMS is a relatively rare syndrome, there is no guidance from controlled studies. Case reports suggest that dantrolene, a skeletal muscle relaxant, and/or bromocriptine, a dopamine agonist, are effective in reducing morbidity and mortality from NMS. There is weak evidence that electroconvulsive therapy is helpful.

### Sedation

Low-potency antipsychotics such as chlorpromazine, clozapine, and quetiapine tend to be more sedating than high-potency agents. However, any antipsychotic can cause some patients to experience sedation. Many patients develop tolerance to this side effect during the first days of treatment. During acute treatment some patients and clinicians may find mild sedation somewhat helpful, particularly when patients are anxious or agitated. If daytime sedation is unpleasant to the patient, taking the antipsychotic at bedtime may be helpful.

### Hypotension

Antipsychotics with alpha-adrenergic effects can cause orthostatic hypotension with associated tachycardia. For a number of commonly prescribed agents, including risperidone, paliperidone, iloperidone, and clozapine, the antipsychotic dose should be titrated and patients and their clinicians should observe for dizziness and other signs of hypotension. For inpatients, iloperidone should be started at 1 mg bid and increased by 1 mg bid each day until a dose of 6 to 12 bid is reached. Clozapine should be started at 12.5 mg bid the first day and increased by 25 to 50 mg daily until patients reach a therapeutic dose. Although hypotension is not as prominent with risperidone, it is usually preferable to start patients at 1 or 2 mg the first day and to increase the dose by 1 or 2 mg if it is well tolerated.

### Metabolic Effects

Metabolic effects of antipsychotics such as weight gain, insulin resistance, and lipid elevation are usually a concern during long-term treatment and will be discussed in detail in Chapter 4. However, some patients experience substantial weight gain during the first weeks of treatment. Moreover, these increases can be associated with the development of insulin resistance. For example, one study (12) found that the administration of olanzapine to healthy, normal-weight men for just 12 days led to substantial increases in food intake, weight, and triglyceride levels. This suggests that clinicians should look for evidence of weight gain and insulin resistance during the first 2 weeks of treatment—particularly when patients are being treated with olanzapine. If this occurs, with olanzapine or other antipsychotics associated with weight gain or metabolic effects, clinicians should reconsider the selection of the antipsychotic.

## Other Side Effects

There are other side effects of antipsychotics that are relatively uncommon, such as endocrine effects and QT prolongation. Since these side effects are more common during long-term treatment, they are discussed in Chapter 4.

## Inpatient Management

The inpatient stay should be viewed as a component of a continuing system of care for the individual with schizophrenia. Although reducing the severity of psychotic symptoms is an important goal, the hospital stay also provides an opportunity for educating the patient and others in the patient's life about schizophrenia, finding a medication regimen that is comfortable for the patient, addressing issues such as housing, vocational, or educational needs, and identifying sources for pharmacological and psychosocial treatments post-discharge. Since there are pressures to keep hospital stays as brief as possible, discharge planning should begin as soon as possible.

## Safety in the Inpatient Setting

Patients who are experiencing an acute psychosis are at an increased risk for dangerous behaviors. Clinicians should regularly assess the contents of a patient's hallucinations and delusions and should directly inquire as to whether the person is having violent or suicidal thoughts. For example, suspicious ideas about a nursing staff member could lead to violent behaviors, or command hallucinations to carry out a self-destructive act could lead to a suicide attempt. In contrast to patients with other illnesses, psychotic individuals who also have a lack of expressiveness (that is, blunted affect) may not demonstrate the emotions that clinicians associate with dangerous behaviors.

## Establishing a Healing Environment

Many individuals with acute schizophrenia complain that they are troubled by excessive stimulation in their environment. They may experience an inability to "filter" extraneous sights and sounds. Moreover, they may misinterpret social signals and may experience dangers in their environment that do not exist. These individuals may benefit from being able to spend time in places on inpatient units that are relatively quiet and not overly stimulating. For similar reasons, group and individual psychotherapies on inpatient units should be relatively non-stressful for patients with psychosis.

## Patient and Family Education

The inpatient hospitalization can provide an opportunity to begin educating patients and their families about schizophrenia and its treatments (13). This initial education can include the patient, or just family members if the patient is reluctant or too ill to participate. This also provides an opportunity for addressing concerns about the patient's medications and the overall treatment plan. This initial interaction with the patient's family may lead to a longer continuing process of family psychoeducation. The Schizophrenia Patient Outcome Research Team (PORT) reviewed the literature on the effectiveness of family psychoeducation, which is discussed in Chapter 4. There is substantial evidence that educational programs for patients and families can improve medication adherence and satisfaction with treatment, as well as illness outcomes. Patients who have substantial contact with their families can benefit from education programs designed for family members. Approaches to the education of families are discussed in Chapter 4.

## Key Points for the Evaluation and Management of Acute Psychosis

- The initial evaluation should include an assessment of potentially dangerous behaviors.
- Command auditory hallucinations can be an important signal of a risk of dangerous behaviors.
- The evaluation should consider possible medical causes of psychosis, including street drugs and prescription medications.
- Physical restraint of agitated patients should only be used as a last resort.
- The selection of an antipsychotic should be guided by concerns about its likely side effects.
- If an individual fails to show any improvement after 2 weeks on an antipsychotic, the selected drug and the dose should be reconsidered.
- Higher doses of antipsychotics are seldom more effective than moderate doses.
- Patients with an acute psychosis are likely to benefit from hospital environments that are not overly stimulating.

## References

1. Singh JP, Grann M, Lichtenstein P, Langstrom N, Fazel S. A novel approach to determining violence risk in schizophrenia: developing a stepped strategy in 13,806 discharged patients. *PLoS One*. 2012;7(2):e31727.

2. Dumais A, Potvin S, Joyal C, Allaire JF, Stip E, Lesage A, et al. Schizophrenia and serious violence: a clinical-profile analysis incorporating impulsivity and substance-use disorders. *Schizophr Res*. 2011;130(1–3):234–237.

3. Suokas JT, Perala J, Suominen K, Saarni S, Lonnqvist J, Suvisaari JM. Epidemiology of suicide attempts among persons with psychotic disorder in the general population. *Schizophr Res*. 2010;124(1–3):22–28.

4. Fazel S, Gulati G, Linsell L, Geddes JR, Grann M. Schizophrenia and violence: systematic review and meta-analysis. *PLoS Med*. 2009;6(8):e1000120.

5. Cheung P, Schweitzer I, Crowley K, Tuckwell V. Violence in schizophrenia: role of hallucinations and delusions. *Schizophr Res*. 1997;26(2–3):181–190.

6. Sikich L, Frazier JA, McClellan J, Findling RL, Vitiello B, Ritz L, et al. Double-blind comparison of first- and second-generation antipsychotics in early-onset schizophrenia and schizo-affective disorder: findings from the treatment of early-onset schizophrenia spectrum disorders (TEOSS) study. *Am J Psychiat*. 2008;165(11):1420–1431.

7. Leucht S, Kissling W, Davis JM. Second-generation antipsychotics for schizophrenia: can we resolve the conflict? *Psychol Med*. 2009;39(10):1591–1602.

8. McEvoy JP, Lieberman JA, Stroup TS, Davis SM, Meltzer HY, Rosenheck RA, et al. Effectiveness of clozapine versus olanzapine, quetiapine, and risperidone in patients with chronic schizophrenia who did not respond to prior atypical antipsychotic treatment. *Am J Psychiat*. 2006;163(4):600–610.

9. Sachdev P, Kruk J. Restlessness: the anatomy of a neuropsychiatric symptom. *Aust N Z J Psychiat*. 1996;30(1):38–53.

10. Gurrera RJ, Caroff SN, Cohen A, Carroll BT, DeRoos F, Francis A, et al. An international consensus study of neuroleptic malignant syndrome diagnostic criteria using the Delphi method. *J Clin Psychiat.* 2011;72(9):1222–1228.

11. Trollor JN, Chen X, Chitty K, Sachdev PS. Comparison of neuroleptic malignant syndrome induced by first- and second-generation antipsychotics. *Br J Psychiat.* 2012;201(1):52–6.

12. Fountaine RJ, Taylor AE, Mancuso JP, Greenway FL, Byerley LO, Smith SR, et al. Increased food intake and energy expenditure following administration of olanzapine to healthy men. *Obesity (Silver Spring).* 2010;18(8):1646–1651.

13. Dixon LB, Dickerson F, Bellack AS, Bennett M, Dickinson D, Goldberg RW, et al. The 2009 schizophrenia PORT psychosocial treatment recommendations and summary statements. *Schizophr Bull.* 2010;36(1):48–70.

# Chapter 3

# Treatment Resistance and the Partial Responder

Patients with schizophrenia vary as to how well they respond to treatment with an antipsychotic. For the best responders, antipsychotics will completely eliminate all of their psychotic symptoms, whereas the worst responders will show little or no improvement. The majority of patients will have responses that are somewhere between; some will have lingering symptoms that minimally interfere with their lives, and others will have symptoms that are a significant burden and require a management strategy. In this chapter, patients who are non-responders or poor responders will be discussed separately from patients who respond well to an antipsychotic, but continue to have persistent psychotic symptoms. These individuals will be referred to as partial responders.

Many patients with mild persistent symptoms will do well without changing their regimen. These individuals can learn to monitor their symptoms and may derive little or no benefit from attempts to eliminate their remaining symptoms.

## Evaluation of Poor Responders

Box 3.1 lists the common causes of a poor response to an antipsychotic. Poor medication adherence may be the most common explanation for a poor antipsychotic response. Among individuals with schizophrenia, nearly half fail to reliably adhere to the prescribed medication regimen (1). The problem is compounded by the reality that psychiatrists tend to severely underestimate the prevalence of non-adherence in the patients they treat. In one study (2), electronic monitoring found poor adherence in 57% of patients, whereas psychiatrists estimated non-adherence at 7%. This suggests that clinicians should consider non-adherence as a cause of a partial response, even when the patient appears to be filling his or her prescriptions. In some cases, carefully reviewing how a patient takes his or her medications can detect missed doses. Asking patients how they deal with the burden of having to take a medication every day can allow patients to reveal adherence problems in an atmosphere that is non-judgmental. In other cases, ordering medication plasma concentrations can be useful in detecting poor adherence.

Substance abuse can also contribute to poor medication responses. Individuals with comorbid substance use disorders can be less engaged in treatment and less adherent (3). Moreover, stimulant drugs such as amphetamine, methamphetamine, and cocaine can worsen schizophrenia and can

**Box 3.1 Contributors to a Poor or Partial Response**

Poor medication adherence
Substance abuse
Inadequate medication levels
Medication side effects

undermine the effects of treatment (4). Many patients and their families view cannabis as a relatively benign drug. However, there is a substantial body of research indicating that cannabis can exacerbate the symptoms of schizophrenia and can result in the rehospitalization of patients (5). In addition, patients who abuse cannabis are more difficult to treat (6).

# When Should a Patient Be Considered a Partial Responder?

Patients should be considered partial responders when they have received an adequate dose of an antipsychotic for a sufficient amount of time. Antipsychotics are usually effective when they are administered at doses that occupy 60%–80% of dopamine $D_2$ receptors (7). There is no indication that higher doses and resulting higher $D_2$ occupancy will result in additional benefit to patients, and higher doses may just increase side effects. Receptor occupancy occurs within a few hours of administering an antipsychotic. However, the reduction in psychotic symptoms may take a few days. Studies suggest that most of the improvement on an antipsychotic occurs within the first 2 weeks after treatment is started (8). If patients fail to show any improvement during this period, it is unlikely that they will respond well to the drug and dose.

These observations suggest important principles for identifying poor and partial responders. Since doses within the usual recommended range will usually result in adequate $D_2$ receptor occupancy, patients should be treated within that range for at least 2 weeks. If an individual shows some improvement in psychosis, it is probably best to continue that dose since improvement often continues during the first month. Patients who show no improvement after 2 weeks are unlikely to show improvement without a change in the regimen.

# First Steps for Non-Responders

There are number of interventions that may be helpful for patients who show no improvement after a period of about 2 weeks. If a patient is not experiencing side effects, increasing the dose within the recommended therapeutic range may be helpful. There is very little clinical evidence to suggest that doses above the range are likely to result in improvements. It is also common for clinicians to add a second antipsychotic or to add an anticonvulsant or mood stabilizer such as lithium, valproate, or carbamazepine in the hope that this will convert a non-responder into a responder. According to the Schizophrenia Patient Outcomes Research Team (PORT) (9), there is inadequate evidence to support these interventions. On the other hand, patients who have mood instability and are excited may benefit from the addition of a mood stabilizer. This may decrease excitement, but is unlikely to decrease the severity of psychosis.

Another alternative is to change the patient to a different antipsychotic medication. This strategy was evaluated in an interesting study (10) that evaluated patients who showed poor responses to 2 weeks of treatment with risperidone. Subjects were then randomized to either staying on risperidone or changing to olanzapine. There was a very small, but statistically significant, advantage for subjects who were changed to olanzapine. The results provide some useful guidance for clinicians in that changing antipsychotics may be somewhat helpful in the absence of a response. However, patients who are poor responders to an adequate trial of an antipsychotic (other than clozapine) are seldom vigorous responders to other antipsychotics. This is not surprising since numerous trials of first- and second-generation antipsychotics—including the National Institute of Mental Health (NIMH) CATIE trial (11)—have usually found that there are no efficacy advantages for any of the antipsychotics, or if there are, the advantages are very small.

## Clozapine for Poor Responders

Patients who respond poorly to first- and second-generation antipsychotics may improve if they are treated with clozapine. This was first demonstrated in a large multicenter trial (12) that carefully characterized patients as treatment refractory (or poor responders) by reviewing their clinical history and by treating them prospectively with haloperidol. When compared with chlorpromazine, clozapine was superior for a broad range of psychopathology, including positive and negative symptoms, as well as anxiety and depression. The results from this study led to the approval of clozapine in the United States for individuals with treatment-refractory schizophrenia. The advantages for clozapine in this population have been reinforced by other trials comparing clozapine to both first- and second-generation antipsychotics. There are other advantages for clozapine in severely ill patients. A large study found an advantage of clozapine over olanzapine for schizophrenia patients with suicidal ideation or suicidal behaviors. This led to the US Food and Drug Administration (FDA) approving clozapine for schizophrenia patients who are at risk for suicide. Other studies (13) suggest that clozapine has advantages for hostility and aggression in treatment-resistant schizophrenia patients.

## Clozapine for Partial Responders

There is also evidence that clozapine can be helpful for schizophrenia patients who are stable, but are burdened by psychotic symptoms. A 29-week study of patients living in the community with partial remissions found that 57% of subjects met stringent improvement criteria with clozapine (14). The strongest evidence may come from the NIMH CATIE study. In that study, subjects who were discontinued from their antipsychotic for a lack of efficacy during Phase 1 were randomly assigned to either clozapine or another second-generation agent (15). Clozapine had clear advantages in that trial. In a study from the United Kingdom (16) patients who were partial responders to antipsychotics were randomized to either clozapine or an antipsychotic selected by their clinician. Again, there were important advantages for clozapine.

Taken together, these studies indicate that patients who are burdened by disturbing psychotic symptoms should receive a clozapine trial. Some clinicians have reserved clozapine for only the most severely ill patients. However, patients who are functioning relatively well in the community may derive substantial benefits if symptoms such as hallucinations or suspiciousness can be reduced. In addition, clinicians who are allowing patients to experience psychotic symptoms for months or even years before treating them with clozapine may be waiting too long. As noted earlier, poor or partial responders can usually be identified after just a few weeks.

## Starting Patients on Clozapine

Prior to starting clozapine, the clinician should assure that there is a system in place for blood monitoring. This requires a system that includes the physician, a laboratory, a pharmacy, and the drug company's clozapine registry. The system should assure that the results of the patient's blood test are sent to the pharmacy, the physician, and the registry.

After obtaining a physical examination, laboratory tests, and an electrocardiogram (ECG), clozapine is started at 12.5 mg administered once or twice the first day and is increased to 25 mg morning and evening the second day. If clozapine is well tolerated, the dose can be increased by 25 mg every other day until a dose of 300 to 450 mg daily is reached. If patients are hospitalized, the titration can be more rapid, with dosage increases of 25 mg daily. In most cases, patients should be dosed two or three times daily, with the larger dose administered before bedtime. Sedation and hypotension are the side effects that may limit dose increases. In nearly all cases, patients will be changing from another antipsychotic to clozapine. The other antipsychotic should be continued until the patient reaches a dose of clozapine that may have therapeutic activity. This is usually approximately 150–200 mg. As patients reach this clozapine dose, the other antipsychotic should be gradually decreased and eventually discontinued. Patients who are able to tolerate a dose of 300–450 mg should continue on that dose for at least an additional 2 weeks. The dose can be increased to as high as 600–900 mg daily if there is inadequate clinical response. Patients should receive clozapine for at least 3 months to determine if this is an effective drug.

Clozapine plasma concentrations can be helpful in decision-making about dosage. A number of studies indicate that patients are more likely to respond when their clozapine plasma levels are greater than 350 ng/ml (17). If the laboratory reports concentrations as clozapine plus norclozapine, levels will be higher. There is no evidence that higher levels than 350 ng/ml are associated with increased effectiveness. A reasonable strategy is for clinicians to monitor plasma concentrations when patients are not showing an adequate response or when side effects are limiting the dose. In these circumstances, the clinician may find that increasing the dose to a level that achieves a plasma level above 350 ng/ml will improve the patient's response.

Patients who are started on clozapine should expect to have side effects. In addition to sedation and hypotension, common side effects are anticholinergic side effects including constipation, difficulty urinating, and blurry vision, low grade fevers, constipation, gastrointestinal discomfort, tachycardia, and sialorrhea. These side effects can be managed in most people. Since constipation can become severe, patients should be warned to increase their fluid intake and to use stool softeners or other treatments at the earliest signs of discomfort.

Patients should also be warned about more serious side effects that can occur early in treatment. Seizures are relatively common during the first weeks of clozapine treatment, and are more common when patients are receiving higher doses. Most of these seizures are tonic-clonic. Patients should probably be warned not to drive during the first weeks of clozapine treatment. In most cases, seizures should not lead to discontinuing clozapine. In the great majority of cases, seizures can be managed by reducing the dose or adding an anticonvulsant such as valproate.

Since clozapine can also be associated with metabolic effects, including weight gain, elevated lipids, and insulin resistance, patients should be told to monitor their weight, and clinicians should monitor lipids and blood glucose.

Clinicians should also be aware that clozapine can cause myocarditis. Although very uncommon, it is also potentially fatal. In the great majority of cases, myocarditis occurs during the first 2 months of clozapine treatment. Early symptoms may include fever (48%), dyspnea (35%), "flu-like illness" (30%), chest pain (22%), and fatigue (17%) (18). The problem is that some of these symptoms are relatively common during the early weeks of clozapine treatment, and they also raise concerns about agranulocytosis. If there is any suspicion of myocarditis, plasma troponin (19) and c-reactive protein (20) levels should be ordered and a cardiologist should be contacted.

## Monitoring for Agranulocytosis

Patients receiving clozapine need to be monitored for evidence that they have or will develop agranulocytosis. Table 3.1 describes the monitoring requirements for prescribing clozapine.

Fortunately, fatalities from agranulocytosis are rare, occurring in as few as.03% of patients treated with clozapine. The risk of agranulocytosis is approximately 0.7%, indicating that the great majority of cases can be managed through early detection. The question that torments many clinicians is when to discontinue clozapine when patients develop neutropenia or when the neutrophil count is dropping. The guidelines require that the clinician discontinue clozapine when the absolute neutrophil count (ANC) is below

## Table 3.1 Frequency of Monitoring Based on Stage of Therapy or Results from WBC and ANC Monitoring Tests

| Situation | Hematological Values for Monitoring | Frequency of WBC and ANC Monitoring |
|---|---|---|
| Initiation of therapy | To initiate therapy WBC should be ≥3500/mm³ and ANC should be ≥2000/mm³<br><br>Note: Do not initiate in patients with history of myeloproliferative disorder or<br><br>Clozarile or clozapine induced agranulocytosis or granulocytopenia | Weekly for 6 months |
| 6–12 months of therapy | Continue if WBC ≥3500/mm³ and ANC ≥2000/mm³ | Every 2 weeks for 6 months |
| 12 months of therapy | Continue if WBC ≥3500/mm³ and ANC ≥2000/mm³ | Every 4 weeks ad infinitum |
| Immature forms present | N/A | Repeat WBC and ANC |
| Discontinuation of therapy | N/A | Weekly for at least 4 weeks from day of discontinuation or until WBC 23500/mm³ and ANC >2000/mm³ |
| Substantial drop in WBC or ANC | Single drop or cumulative drop within 3 weeks of WBC ≥3000/mm³ and ANC ≥1500/mm³ | 1. Repeat WBC and ANC<br>2. If repeat values are WBC 3000–3500/mm³ and ANC >2000/mm³, then monitor twice weekly |
| Mild leukopenia, mild granulocytopenia | If WBC 3000–3500/mm³ and/or ANC 1500–2000/mm³ | Twice-weekly until WBC >3500/mm³ and ANC >2000/mm³ then return to previous monitoring frequency |
| Moderate leukopenia and/or moderate granulocytopenia | If WBC 2000–3000/mm³ and/or ANC 1000–1500/mm³ | 1. Interrupt therapy<br>2. Monitor daily until WBC >3000/mm³ and ANC >2000/mm³<br>3. Monitor twice weekly until WBC >3500/mm³ and ANC >2000/mm³<br>4. May rechallenge when WBC >3500/mm³ and ANC >2000/mm³<br>5. If rechallenged monitor weekly for 1 year before returning to the usual monitoring schedule. |

*(Continued)*

| Situation | Hematological Values for Monitoring | Frequency of WBC and ANC Monitoring |
|---|---|---|
| Severe leukopenia and/or severe granulocytopenia | If WBC <2000/mm³ and/or ANC <1000/mm³ | Discontinue treatment and do not rechallenge patient |
| | | Monitor until normal and for at least 4 weeks from day of discontinuation as follows: |
| | | Daily until WBC >3000/mm³ and ANC >1500/mm³ |
| | | Twice weekly until WBC >3500/mm³ and ANC >2000/mm³ |
| | | Weekly after WBC >3500/mm³ |
| Agranulocytosis | ANC 500/mm³ | Discontinue treatment and do not rechallenge patient |
| | | Monitor until normal and for at least 4 weeks from day of discontinuation as follows: |
| | | Daily until \WBC >3000/mm³ and ANC >1500/mm³ |
| | | Twice weekly until WBC >3500/mm³ and ANC >2000/mm³ |
| | | Weekly after WBC >3500/mm³ |

WBC = white blood cell count; ANC = absolute neutrophil count

1000/mm³ or when the white blood count is below 2000/mm³. Under these conditions, clozapine cannot be restarted. If the ANC is between 1000 and 1500, clozapine should be stopped, but it can be restarted when the ANC is above 1500. For some patients—particularly those of Middle Eastern or African descent—it is common for the ANC to drop below 1500, with or without clozapine. As a result, clozapine treatment can be particularly challenging with occasional interruptions. Clinicians should also be aware that some patients tend to have lower ANCs in the morning. Moving the blood draws to later in the day can be helpful for these individuals.

## Managing Partial Responders to Clozapine

It is not uncommon for patients to improve on clozapine, but nevertheless continue to experience psychotic symptoms. A number of studies have explored adding a low dose of a high-potency antipsychotic. Most of these studies added risperidone. A meta-analysis of studies that added a second antipsychotic to clozapine (21) found that open label studies tended to favor adding a second antipsychotic, but double-blind studies did not find statistically significant effects.

Nevertheless, a close look at the risperidone studies suggests that there were positive effects in some patients. As a result, this may be a useful intervention when patients continue to experience disturbing symptoms on clozapine. If patients fail to improve, the second antipsychotic can be discontinued.

## Electroconvulsive Therapy

Another approach for partial responders who fail to improve on clozapine or other antipsychotics is to add electroconvulsive therapy (ECT). Studies in this area include mostly case reports that tend to be biased in favor of positive reports. Nevertheless, a recent meta-analysis (22) concluded that ECT was a reasonable option when pharmacotherapy was insufficient for treating psychosis. Patients who are partial responders to clozapine have also shown improvement with the addition of ECT.

## Cognitive Behavioral Treatment for Partial Responders

Patients who have persisting psychotic symptoms may also improve with cognitive behavioral therapy (CBT) for psychosis. This is a specialized form of CBT that addresses positive symptoms by having patients question the evidence that led to their hallucinations or their irrational beliefs. The CBT therapist guides the patient through a process that revisits the development of the patient's symptoms and eventually leads to cognitive restructuring to correct the cognitive processes that led to the symptom (19–23). This can result in a clinically meaningful reduction in the patient's symptom burden.

A number of studies from the United Kingdom support the effectiveness of CBT for psychosis. As a result, it is considered to be a preferred practice. It has also gained acceptance in the United States and is considered an evidence-based practice in the Schizophrenia PORT (Patient Outcome Research Team). Although most well-controlled studies have found positive results, the effect sizes have varied. There is also evidence that the improvements from CBT tend to persist after the treatment is completed (20–24).

CBT is an option that should be considered for patients who have persistent psychotic symptoms after an adequate trial on an antipsychotic. These include patients who continue to have disturbing symptoms on clozapine. The best candidates for CBT for psychosis are willing to explore the origin of their symptoms. There are different forms of CBT, and training manuals for each are available. Studies suggest that the effects of CBT are more likely to endure if patients receive at least 10 sessions over 6 months (21–25).

## Assertive Community Treatments for Poor Responders

Assertive community treatment (ACT) is a strategy for managing seriously mentally ill patients who are high utilizers of expensive services such as hospitalization and homeless services. These services are commonly provided in public mental health settings such as community mental health centers and VA clinics. The components of ACT include a multidisciplinary treatment team that is always available if a patient is in crisis. Early studies found that ACT reduces the need for hospitalization and improves community adjustment (26). Moreover, the intervention was cost effective (27). A recent Cochrane review (28) confirmed that ACT reduced the need for hospitalization and improved the likelihood of independent living. The advantages for reducing the overall cost of treatment were less clear. On the other hand, patients receiving ACT were more likely to remain in contact with services. A study from the VA (29) found that ACT was also associated with increased adherence with antipsychotics.

ACT teams have been widely disseminated in the United States in public health systems and in the VA. They have also been successfully implemented outside the United States. Individuals with persistent symptoms of psychosis who are high utilizers of services such as hospitals and emergency rooms should be considered for ACT programs. The components of ACT teams are listed in Box 3.2.

---

**Box 3.2  Components of ACT Teams**

• Team is mobile and provides most services in the community.
• A multidisciplinary team organizes and delivers comprehensive services to patients in a timely and integrated fashion.
• High staff-to-patient ratio, e.g., 1:10 or 1:12.
• Services are available 24 hours, 7 days.

---

## Key Points for Treatment Resistance and the Poor Responder

•  Before considering someone a poor responder, consider poor medication adherence, substance use, inadequate drug levels, and side effects.
•  Frequently used interventions such as high doses, mood stabilizers, and antipsychotic polypharmacy are seldom effective for poor responders.
•  Patients should not be considered poor or partial responders until they have an adequate trial of clozapine
•  Cognitive behavioral treatment for psychosis can reduce the severity of psychotic symptoms.
•  Patients who are high utilizers of hospitals and emergency rooms should be considered for assertive community treatment

## References

1. Lacro JP, et al. Prevalence of and risk factors for medication nonadherence in patients with schizophrenia: a comprehensive review of recent literature. *J Clin Psychiat.* 2002;63(10):892–909.

2. Byerly MJ et al. Validity of electronically monitored medication adherence and conventional adherence measures in schizophrenia. *Psychiatr Serv.* 2007;58(6):844–847.

3. Stowkowy J, et al. Predictors of disengagement from treatment in an early psychosis program. *Schizophr Res.* 2012;136(1–3):7–12.

4. Green AI. Schizophrenia and comorbid substance use disorder: effects of antipsychotics. *J Clin Psychiat.* 2005;66(suppl 6):21–26.

5. van Dijk D, et al. Effect of cannabis use on the course of schizophrenia in male patients: a prospective cohort study. *Schizophr Res.* 2012;137(1–3):50–57.

6. Leeson VC, et al. The effect of cannabis use and cognitive reserve on age at onset and psychosis outcomes in first-episode schizophrenia. *Schizophr Bull.* 2012;38(4):873–880.

7. Seeman P. Dopamine D2 receptors as treatment targets in schizophrenia. *Clin Schizophr Relat Psychoses.* 2010;4(1):56–73.

8. Suzuki T, et al. Time course of improvement with antipsychotic medication in treatment-resistant schizophrenia. *Br J Psychiat.* 2011;199(4):275–280.

9. Buchanan RW, et al. The 2009 schizophrenia PORT psychopharmacological treatment recommendations and summary statements. *Schizophr Bull.* 2010;36(1):71–93.

10. Kinon BJ, et al. Early response to antipsychotic drug therapy as a clinical marker of subsequent response in the treatment of schizophrenia. *Neuropsychopharmacol.* 2010;35(2):581–590.

11. Lieberman JA, et al. Effectiveness of antipsychotic drugs in patients with chronic schizophrenia. *N Engl J Med.* 2005;353(12):1209–1223.

12. Kane JM, et al. Clozapine for the treatment-resistant schizophrenic: a double-blind comparison versus chlorpromazine/benztropine. *Arch Gen Psychiat.* 1988. 45(789–796).

13. Volavka J, Citrome L. Pathways to aggression in schizophrenia affect results of treatment. *Schizophr Bull.* 2011;37(5):921–929.

14. Kane JM, et al. Clozapine and haloperidol in moderately refractory schizophrenia: a 6-month randomized and double-blind comparison. *Arch Gen Psychiat.* 2001;58(10):965–972.

15. McEvoy JP, et al. Effectiveness of clozapine versus olanzapine, quetiapine, and risperidone in patients with chronic schizophrenia who did not respond to prior atypical antipsychotic treatment. *Am J Psychiat.* 2006;163(4):600–610.

16. Lewis SW, et al. Randomized controlled trial of effect of prescription of clozapine versus other second-generation antipsychotic drugs in resistant schizophrenia. *Schizophr Bull.* 2006;32(4):715–723.

17. Miller DD, et al. Plasma clozapine concentrations as a predictor of clinical response: a follow-up study. *J Clin Psychiat.* 1994;55(suppl B):117–121.

18. Merrill DB, Dec GW, Goff DC. Adverse cardiac effects associated with clozapine. *J Clin Psychopharmacol.* 2005;25(1):32–41.

19. Marder SR, et al. Physical health monitoring of patients with schizophrenia. *Am J Psychiat.* 2004;161(8):1334–1349.

20. Ronaldson KJ, et al. A new monitoring protocol for clozapine-induced myocarditis based on an analysis of 75 cases and 94 controls. *Aust N Z J Psychiat.* 2011;45(6):458–465.

21. Barbui C, et al. Does the addition of a second antipsychotic drug improve clozapine treatment? *Schizophr Bull.* 2009;35(2):458–468.

22. Pompili M, et al. Indications for electroconvulsive treatment in schizophrenia: a systematic review. *Schizophr Res.* 2013;146(1–3):1–9.

23. Beck AT, Rector NA. Cognitive therapy of schizophrenia: a new therapy for the new millennium. *Am J Psychother.* 2000;54(3):291–300.

24. Turkington D, et al. A randomized controlled trial of cognitive-behavior therapy for persistent symptoms in schizophrenia: a five-year follow-up. *Schizophr Res.* 2008;98(1–3):1–7.

25. Turkington D, Kingdon D, Chadwick P. Cognitive-behavioural therapy for schizophrenia: filling the therapeutic vacuum. *Br J Psychiat.* 2003;183:98–99.

26. Stein LI, Test MA. Alternative to mental hospital treatment. I. Conceptual model, treatment program, and clinical evaluation. *Arch Gen Psychiat.* 1980;37(4):392–397.

27. Weisbrod BA, Test AM, Stein LI. Alternative to mental hospital treatment. II. Economic benefit-cost analysis. *Arch Gen Psychiat.* 1980;37(4):400–405.

28. Marshall M, Lockwood A. Assertive community treatment for people with severe mental disorders. *Cochrane Database Syst Rev.*2000;2:CD001089.

29. Valenstein M, et al. Assertive community treatment in veterans affairs settings: impact on adherence to antipsychotic medication. *Psychiatr Serv.* 2013;64(5):445–451

# Chapter 4

# The Stable Phase and Recovery

The great majority of patients with schizophrenia who receive an antipsychotic will spend most of their lives in a stable state. The amount of symptom burden among stable patients will vary, with some achieving a complete remission while others continue to experience symptoms that may impair the quality of their lives. For many patients, positive symptoms will be mild and usually well tolerated. However, negative symptoms and cognitive impairments, as well as depression and anxiety, may affect their overall adjustment in the community. The goals of treatment during this phase of treatment are to prevent patients from suffering a relapse in their psychotic symptoms, to manage symptoms that persist, and to assist patients in meeting their own goals.

## Recovery in Schizophrenia

Clinicians who treat schizophrenia should set goals that are more ambitious than merely preventing relapse. Patients and their families are interested in improving the functioning of patients as well as their quality of life. This more ambitious approach has been characterized as an orientation toward "recovery" (2). Unfortunately, there has been considerable confusion about the definition of "recovery," with some rejecting the term under the assumption that it refers a goal that is not reachable for most patients. For the purposes of this chapter, recovery will refer to an approach to treatment that emphasizes the patient setting his or her goals. These goals may include living more independently, succeeding at school or work, or improving social relationships. Recovery-oriented treatment also conveys optimism. It emphasizes that individuals with schizophrenia may improve the quality of their lives, even when patients continue to be burdened by symptoms of their illness. As will be noted in the following sections, there is evidence that recovery is promoted by the judicious combining of antipsychotic medications and psychosocial treatments.

## Antipsychotics During the Stable Phase

There is a large body of evidence indicating that antipsychotic medications are effective for reducing the risk that patients will experience a psychotic relapse (3, 4). Most of the studies used a similar design. Patients who had been stabilized on an antipsychotic medication were randomly assigned to receive an antipsychotic or a placebo. The main outcome measure is the risk of experiencing a psychotic relapse. The results from studies are remarkably consistent. Approximately 64% of patients who are changed to a placebo will relapse, compared with only 27% of patients who receive an antipsychotic. The rate of relapse will be lower if patients are guaranteed drug delivery with a depot antipsychotic. Many clinicians have wondered if the risk of stopping an antipsychotic is lower for patients who have been well and stable for long periods of time. This was examined by studies that evaluated the risk of relapse in patients who had been stable for prolonged periods of time (5). The risk of discontinuing antipsychotics in these individuals was similar to the risk in studies of other multiple-episode patients.

There are other advantages for maintaining patients on antipsychotics. Psychotic relapses that occur in patients who are receiving an antipsychotic tend to be less severe than those in patients who are not receiving medication. The lower severity is manifest in fewer assaultive episodes and suicide attempts, as well as fewer involuntary hospitalizations (6).

This body of evidence provides guidance for clinical practice. The great majority of patients with schizophrenia should continue on an antipsychotic after they have recovered from a psychotic relapse. In many cases it can be difficult to explain to patients that it is important to stay on their medication when they are symptom-free. This is especially difficult when patients are experiencing side effects from their medications.

## Managing Non-adherence

The most common cause of relapse in schizophrenia is medication non-adherence (7). Unfortunately, non-adherence is common; a Veterans Affairs study found that 61% of schizophrenia patients had adherence problems at some time during a 4-year period (8). In addition to higher rates of relapse and rehospitalization, non-adherence is also associated with a worse functional outcome (9).

Clinicians tend to underestimate the levels of non-adherence in their patients. This may result from the reluctance of many patients to admit to their provider that they are not following their directions and from a tendency of many clinicians to not actively monitor medication adherence. Barry Blackwell (10) has noted that just asking patients if they are taking their medications may elicit a defensive response if the patient believes that he or she will be criticized by the provider. He suggests the alternative of asking about the difficulties of taking medication once or more a day in a manner that is not judgmental and which may provide an opportunity for patients to discuss their attitudes toward taking antipsychotics.

## Oral and Long-Acting Antipsychotics

Both oral and long-acting injectable antipsychotics (LAIs) are effective for stable phase treatment. Studies comparing the effectiveness of oral and depot antipsychotics have yielded confusing results. Open-label studies have tended to find substantial advantages for long-acting medications. Although meta-analyses of controlled trials have tended to show advantages for LAIs, the trials are inconsistent and the differences tend to be modest (11, 12). On the other hand, there are reasons to believe that the well-controlled studies may underestimate the advantages of LAIs. The most important reason is that the patients who are most likely to benefit from LAIs are unlikely to be represented in these studies. That is, the advantages may be most apparent in patients with more severe illnesses, who are less cooperative. These individuals are commonly excluded from research studies. In addition, the monitoring that tends to occur in these trials usually exceeds the clinical interactions in most settings. Infrequent monitoring of patients receiving oral medications may lead to irregular pill taking.

Although it is unclear if LAIs are superior in clinical trials, there are large groups of patients who clearly benefit from this route of administration. These groups include patients who are unreliable pill takers, those who have a history of relapse due to non-adherence with oral medications, and patients who acknowledge that it is easier to receive an injection than take pills daily.

Another advantage of LAIs is that they may have milder side effects in some patients. The reason is that patients who receive an oral antipsychotic usually have a higher maximum plasma concentration (Cmax) than patients who receive an LAI (13). Since some side effects are related to Cmax, patients may tolerate the LAI better than the oral compound.

## Changing Patients to a Long-Acting Injectable Antipsychotic

There are a number of considerations when changing patients from an oral antipsychotic to an LAI (14). First, the LAI is 100% bioavailable. In contrast, oral compounds may be extensively metabolized in the liver and the gut. As a result, clinicians should be cautious in translating the optimal dose of the oral antipsychotic into a corresponding dose of the LAI. The other important consideration is that it may take a substantial amount of time for a patient to reach a steady-state plasma after they are changed to an LAI. In many cases, patients will require as long as 3 months. During these months, the patient may not have a sufficient plasma concentration of the drug for preventing relapse. However, even if the clinician continues the same dose, the patient may have a gradually increasing plasma level. Moreover, if the clinician increases the dose during this period, the patient may experience side effects that are difficult to manage because a reduction does not immediately result in a reduced drug level.

These considerations point to a very reasonable strategy for patients who are being changed from an oral to a long-acting antipsychotic. In most cases, patients should have a cross titration from the oral to the depot drug. That is, the LAI should be started at a low to moderate dose and continued at that dose if it is well tolerated. The oral antipsychotic should be continued, but the dose should be gradually decreased over the next 2 to 3 months and eventually discontinued. Adjustments to the depot dose should be made when the blood level is at or near steady state. A possible exception to this strategy may be appropriate for the patient who is being started on paliperidone palmitate or olanzapine pamoate. Following an injection of these LAIs, there is a sufficient release of paliperidone or olanzapine to provide antipsychotic activity.

## Considerations in Selecting an LAI

Table 4.1 lists the LAIs that are available in the United States. Factors to consider are the intervals between injections, the costs of the agents, and their potential side effects. At this time there is no indication that there are differences in efficacy among the available LAIs. The side effects of these agents resemble those of the corresponding oral agents. Occasionally, patients will experience injection site reactions with pain and redness.

Following are special concerns for patients receiving one of the newer LAIs:

- *Risperidone microspheres* should be administered every 2 weeks at doses of 12.5 to 50 mg. The formulation requires refrigeration and the mixing of ingredients immediately prior to IM administration.

### Table 4.1 Long-Acting Injectable Antipsychotic Medications (LAIs)

| | Dose Range (mg) | Injection Interval | Available Doses | Notes |
|---|---|---|---|---|
| Fluphenazine decanoate | 12.5–100 mg | 2–4 weeks | 25 mg/ml vials | z-track injection in gluteal or deltoid |
| Haloperidol decanoate | 50–200 mg | 4 weeks | 50 or 100 mg/ml vials | z-track injection in gluteal or deltoid |
| Risperidone microspheres | 12.5–50 mg | 2 weeks | 12.5, 25, 37.5 or 50 mg | Requires storage in a refrigerator |
| Paliperidone palmitate | 39–234 mg | 4 weeks | 39, 78, 117, 156, or 234 mg | |
| Olanzapine pamoate | 150–405 mg | 2–4 weeks | 210, 300, or 405 mg | Patients should be observed for 3 hours after each injection for post-injection delirium sedation |
| Aripiprazole extended-release suspension | 200–400 mg | 4 weeks | 300 and 400 mg | Reduce dose for cyp2D6 poor metabolizers |

- *Olanzapine pamoate* has the potential for causing a post-injection delirium sedation syndrome following an injection. This reaction is uncommon but serious in that patients can experience dizziness, confusion, disorientation, and excessive sedation. As a result, patients should be observed by a health care professional for 3 hours after each injection. Sites that administer long-acting olanzapine need to be registered before administering the drug. The recommended doses are 150–300 mg every 2 weeks or 405 mg every 4 weeks.
- *Paliperidone palmitate* is released on the first day following an injection. As a result, patients who are unable to take oral medications can be changed without a cross-titration period. A higher maximum plasma concentration is reached when the drug is injected into the deltoid rather than the gluteal muscle. Therefore, if a clinician is starting a patient on paliperidone palmitate without a cross-titration from an oral antipsychotic, deltoid administration may be preferred. On the other hand, if minimal side effects are a priority, gluteal administration has advantages. Most patients can be managed with doses from 117 to 234 mg every 4 weeks.
- *Aripiprazole monohydrate* is slowly absorbed, with a time to maximum plasma concentration of about 5 to 7 days and a mean terminal elimination half-life of 29.9 days for the 300 mg dose and 46.5 days for 400 mg. Steady state is reached after 4 injections. As a result, the patient's oral antipsychotic should be continued for at least 14 days.

## Discontinuing Antipsychotics

Most patients with schizophrenia should be continued on their antipsychotics indefinitely. However, there are some circumstances where a decision is made to discontinue antipsychotics. These include patients who insist on having their medications discontinued, despite the recommendations of their clinicians and others, or when there is agreement that a trial off medications is reasonable. The decision to discontinue antipsychotics should be carefully discussed with the patient and others who are close to the patient. It is particularly important that the patient understand that remaining stable during the first weeks or months following drug discontinuation is not evidence that medications are not necessary. Studies have suggested that the majority of relapses occur more than 4 months after drugs are stopped (4). This suggests that patients should continue to be monitored by a provider who can resume an antipsychotic if there is evidence that the patient is relapsing.

If a decision is made to discontinue antipsychotics, the patient and the clinician should develop a strategy for detecting early warning or prodromal signs of impending relapse. For most patients, psychotic relapse does not occur abruptly. Rather, there is a period of weeks or months during which patients show evidence that they are worsening (15). Since the warning signs for an individual tend to be the same for each episode, it can be useful to review these episodes with patients and their family members. A number of studies have evaluated early intervention strategies as a means of minimizing the amount of time that patients are treated with an antipsychotic. Antipsychotics are discontinued between episodes, and patients are treated when they show early signs of relapse. Although this strategy has not been shown to be as effective as continuous drug treatment, there are individuals who tend to avoid serious relapses with this approach (16, 17).

## Symptoms During the Stable Phase

During the stable phase, psychotic symptoms can often be controlled or eliminated. However, other symptoms will commonly affect the patient's overall adjustment. As noted below, these symptoms are seldom responsive to antipsychotic medications and may require specific management strategies.

### Negative Symptoms

The negative symptoms of schizophrenia are characterized by an absence or reduction in behaviors and functions that are normally present. A National Institute of Mental Health (NIMH) consensus meeting proposed blunted affect, anhedonia, alogia, asociality, and avolition as key negative symptom domains (18). The result of these symptoms is commonly a loss of motivation and goal-directed behavior and marked impairments in functioning and quality of life. A recent analysis of a large trial found that negative symptoms had a greater impact on functional outcomes than positive symptoms (19). Negative symptoms are common in both first-episode patients (20) and stabilized multi-episode patients. The prevalence varies depending on the criteria, but an overview of the literature suggests that approximately 40% of patients have prominent negative symptoms (21).

Common negative symptoms of schizophrenia include the following:

- *Blunted or restricted affect*: Includes a lack of facial expressiveness and use of expressive gestures.
- *Anhedonia*: A decreased ability to experience pleasure. Recent research (22) suggests that negative symptom patients have a decreased ability to anticipate reward.
- *Alogia*: Decreased speech
- *Asociality*: Diminished interest in social behavior
- *Avolition*: Lack of goal-directed behavior.

In assessing negative symptoms, it is important to separate primary from secondary negative symptoms. In general, primary negative symptoms persist through all stages of the illness. Secondary negative symptoms can result from psychotic symptoms. For example, suspiciousness can lead to a lack of social interaction, and hallucinations can distract patients and decrease goal-directed behaviors. Side effects of antipsychotics, particularly parkinsonian side effects, can lead patients to show decreased expressiveness. Depression—which is also common in schizophrenia—can lead to motor retardation and anhedonia. Depression and negative symptoms can be difficult to discriminate. It can be helpful to note that negative-symptom patients seldom describe themselves as sad.

Aaron Beck and his coworkers (23) have developed an interesting cognitive model of negative symptoms. In this model, patients with negative symptoms have been discouraged by their failures and have developed defeatist beliefs. The presence of defeatist beliefs in negative-symptom patients has been confirmed by other researchers (24) and, as noted below, forms the basis for a treatment approach.

## Managing Negative Symptoms

At the present time there are no evidence-based treatments for negative symptoms. Although antipsychotic medications may be helpful for negative symptoms that are secondary to positive symptoms, they are seldom effective for persistent primary negative symptoms. A number of studies have evaluated antidepressant medications for negative symptoms. Reviews of these trials (25) found that antidepressants tended to have modest effects for improving negative symptoms. There is insufficient information to support any individual antidepressant. This supports the reasonable practice of prescribing an antidepressant such as a selective serotonin reuptake inhibitor (SSRI) for patients with primary negative symptoms. If the additional medication is ineffective, it should be discontinued. Trials of stimulants, modafinil, armodafinil, and other medication have had mixed results (26).

There is some promise that medications currently in development will be effective for negative symptoms. A number of trials of medications with different molecular targets—including glutamate and nicotinic cholinergic receptors—have shown positive results for negative symptoms. These medications would be added to the patient's antipsychotic. Other promising approaches include devices using magnetic stimulation or direct current stimulation.

As mentioned previously, there are promising psychosocial approaches for treating patients with primary negative symptoms. There is evidence that social skills training and cognitive behavioral therapy—described later in this chapter—improve negative symptoms (27). Grant et al. (23) found that a cognitive therapy approach that addressed defeatist beliefs improved negative symptoms as well as functioning.

Taken together, this information suggests that even though there is not a well-supported evidence-based pharmacological or non-pharmacological treatment for negative symptoms, viable options for clinicians to consider include antidepressants, social skills training, and cognitive behavioral therapy.

## Cognitive Impairments

Impaired cognition is a core feature of schizophrenia. When individuals with schizophrenia are administered neuropsychological tests, they tend to perform one to two standard deviations below community samples. This impairment is not limited to a specific cognitive domain but appears to be generalized over multiple domains (28). Speed of processing and impairments in social cognition best distinguish individuals with schizophrenia from unaffected community residents (29). Nearly every individual with schizophrenia has some impairment. For example, individuals with schizophrenia who perform in the normal range on neuropsychological tests tend to have siblings and parents who perform better than average.

It can be helpful to separate cognitive impairments into those domains that are related to social interactions—or social cognition—from impairments in basic cognition. Social cognition encompasses the processes that individuals use for social interactions and includes recognizing the emotions that people express through their faces and their expressive gestures, understanding the intentions of others, perceiving sarcasm, and being able to empathize with others. These functions are severely impaired in many people with schizophrenia and contribute to impaired community functioning (24).

The cognitive domains that are commonly affected in schizophrenia include the following:

- Processing speed
- Attention
- Working memory
- Verbal learning and memory
- Visual learning and memory
- Reasoning/executive functioning
- Verbal comprehension
- Social cognition.

Impairments are usually present at the time of the first episode and have also been found in individuals in the at-risk or prodromal state. The severity of the cognitive deficits is similar in first-episode and multi-episode patients, indicating that schizophrenia is not a dementing illness. The deficits are clinically important since their severity is strongly related to a patient's community functioning and his or her ability to benefit from psychiatric rehabilitation (30).

The severity of cognitive impairments can be difficult to assess without neuropsychological tests. Patients can be relatively poor reporters of their own cognitive abilities, which suggests that clinician interviews may have limited usefulness. Students or people with cognitively demanding work and schizophrenia may be aware of their cognitive limitations. For some patients, other informants, including close relatives or caretakers, may be helping in assessing cognition.

## Treating Cognitive Impairments

Given the strong association of cognitive impairments with functioning, it is plausible that improving cognition will lead to functional gains. Unfortunately, antipsychotic medications are relatively ineffective for improving cognition. The early hope that second-generation antipsychotics would be more effective than first-generation agents has not been substantiated. Other agents, including donepezil, stimulants, modafanil, and galantamine, have been added to antipsychotics in the hope that they would improve cognition. None of them has proven to be effective.

There is evidence that cognitive training or cognitive remediation may be helpful for treating cognitive impairments. A number of approaches have been developed, and all of them include training individuals in a manner that compensates for their impaired cognition or repairs their cognition. All of them include repeated exercises, and nearly all are computer-based. Some interventions are delivered in groups, whereas others are administered to individuals. The availability of web-based programs has made it feasible for patients to self-administer some programs in their homes. Although the different programs for cognitive training vary in their content, meta-analysis indicates that these programs are effective for improving cognition and community functioning. In addition, the effects of cognitive training on functioning are most apparent when it is combined with psychiatric rehabilitation (31).

## Depression in Schizophrenia

Stable patients with schizophrenia often experience symptoms of depression. These symptoms are common, affecting about a third of stable patients (32). The clinical picture resembles that of major depression, with symptoms such as sadness, loss of self-esteem, hopelessness, and anhedonia. It can be associated with relapse, rehospitalization, and a risk of suicide. In evaluating these symptoms, clinicians should rule out other causes of depression such as antipsychotic side effects and negative symptoms. If the depressed mood is associated with parkinsonian side effects or akathisia, a reduction in the antipsychotic dose or the addition of an anticholinergic or propranolol may be helpful. If patients present with apathy and anhedonia and without sadness, this may indicate that negative symptoms are the cause. Depression can also be associated with a recurrence of psychotic sympotms. If this is the case, re-evaluating the antipsychotic and managing the psychosis may be effective for reducing depression.

## Treatment of Depression in Schizophrenia

A number of studies have evaluated the effectiveness of antidepressants for depression in schizophrenia. Overall, the evidence for antidepressants is relatively weak (33). However, this area has not been adequately studied, and there are few alternatives for managing depression. As a result, an antidepressant such as an SSRI is a reasonable intervention. There is very little evidence suggesting that these medications are likely to worsen the patient's psychosis. Although cognitive behavior therapy may be effective for depression symptoms, it has not been adequately studied.

## Side Effects During Stable Phase Treatment

Side effects that are a concern during the first days of treatment with an antipsychotic, including acute extrapyramidal side effects (EPS), sedation, and hypotension, are discussed in Chapter 2. This chapter will focus on the side effects that become a concern during longer term treatment.

# Metabolic Side Effects

Schizophrenia patients are more vulnerable than the general population to illnesses such as coronary heart disease, Type II diabetes mellitus, and hypertension. These illnesses are the largest contributors to the 20% reduction in life expectancy that is associated with schizophrenia (34). Although antipsychotics can be an important contributor to the increased vulnerability for cardiovascular disease, it is important to note that there are other important risk factors in schizophrenia patients, including high rates of smoking, obesity, a sedentary lifestyle, and poor diets.

Given these serious health concerns, individuals with schizophrenia should be considered—as a group—as having a high cardiac risk. This elevated risk should influence the selection of an antipsychotic, as well as the plan for monitoring risk factors. Table 4.2 shows the tendency of different antipsychotics for increasing weight and elevating lipids. If cardiovascular risk is a concern for an individual patient—and in most cases it will be—then olanzapine, quetiapine, and clozapine are likely to make management more difficult. One approach to determining metabolic risk is to assess whether a patient meets the criteria for the metabolic syndrome. Table 4.3 lists the risk factors for the metabolic syndrome. Individuals who meet these criteria should be considered as being in a group with substantially elevated risk (35). On the other hand, individuals who do not meet these criteria may have individual risk factors such as obesity or lipid elevations that can also increase their cardiovascular risk. Finally, younger patients who are treated with some antipsychotics have an even greater vulnerability to weight gain and lipid elevations. For example, in one study of children and adolescents (36), the olanzapine arm of a randomized trial was eliminated from the trial since the metabolic changes were sufficiently severe that including this drug was considered unethical.

## Table 4.2 Metabolic Effects of Commonly Prescribed Antipsychotics

| Antipsychotic | Weight Gain | Lipid Elevations |
|---|---|---|
| Chlorpromazine | +++ | +++ |
| Haloperidol | + | + |
| Perphenazine | ++ | + |
| Clozapine | +++ | +++ |
| Risperidone | ++ | + |
| Olanzapine | +++ | +++ |
| Quetiapine | ++ | +++ |
| ziprasidone | - | - |
| aripiprazole | - | - |
| paliperidone | ++ | + |
| asenapine | + | - |
| iloperidone | ++ | ++ |
| lurasidone | - | - |

- none, + mild, ++ moderate, +++ severe

## Table 4.3 Working Criteria for the Metabolic Syndrome

|  | ATP-III-A (3/5 criteria required) |
|---|---|
| Waist (cm) | M>102, F>88 |
| Blood pressure (mm/Hg) | ≥130/85* |
| HDL (mg/dl) | M<40, F<50 |
| Triglycerides (mg/dl) | ≥150 |
| Glucose (mg/dl) | ≥100** |

*Abbreviations*: ATP, Adult Treatment Panel[36]; ATP-A, Adult Treatment Protocol-Adapted[37]; IDF, International Diabetes Federation[38]; M, males; F, females; HDL, high density lipoproteins; *or treated with antihypertensive medication; **or treated with insulin or hypoglycemic medication.

# Managing Cardiovascular Risk in Schizophrenia

Managing this risk should be a component of the long-term treatment strategy. Conferences at Mount Sinai Medical Center (34), as well as the American Diabetes Association and the American Psychiatric Association (37), have each proposed guidelines for the routine monitoring of metabolic risk factors. These guidelines are all relatively similar and include the regular monitoring of weight, glucose, and lipids. The Mount Sinai recommendations are included in Table 4.4. Implementing metabolic monitoring may be difficult in some settings. For example, many prescribers do not have access to a scale and blood pressure cuffs. This can be addressed by asking patients to weigh themselves and to measure their own blood pressure.

Clinicians who are interested in safely administering olanzapine, quetiapine, or clozapine may also consider more frequent monitoring. For example, patients receiving these medications would be urged to weigh themselves on a regular basis and to contact the prescriber if weight gain meets a particular threshold. Although weight is the easiest parameter to measure, some individuals may show evidence of insulin resistance without weight gain. This can be addressed by measuring triglyceride levels before and 4 to 8 weeks after starting the drug. An increase in triglycerides may indicate increasing insulin resistance (38). Since insulin resistance is an independent risk factor for cardiovascular disease and the development of Type II diabetes, the clinician may decide that there is a need for an intervention.

## Table 4.4 Metabolic Monitoring Guidelines from Mount Sinai Conference

| Body mass index or weight | BMI at baseline; at every visit for next 6 months; quarterly when stable |
|---|---|
| Plasma glucose | Fasting plasma glucose or HbA1c before initiating an antipsychotic, annually thereafter |
| Lipid panel | Yearly if levels are in the normal range and every 6 months if LDL levels are >130mg/dL |

# Managing Metabolic Risk

*Switching to an antipsychotic with a lower liability for metabolic effects*: The decision about how much weight gain should be tolerated before an intervention, and what the intervention should be, can be made jointly by a patient and his or her clinician. If the weight gain is clearly related to an antipsychotic, changing the antipsychotic had been shown to be an effective intervention. For example, the NIMH CATIE (39) study found that patients who gained weight during the first phase were likely to lose weight and show improvement on other metabolic measures when they were changed to ziprasidone. Another large study (40) found similar results when patients were changed to aripiprazole.

Many patients will not be candidates for switching antipsychotics. The patient may prefer the drug associated with weight gain, or the individual may have failed trials with other medications. In these cases, there are other approaches to limiting the metabolic effects.

*Psychosocial approaches to weight management*: A number of individual and group-based programs have been developed for helping patients to address metabolic problems through diet and exercise (41). These included approaches that focused on preventing weight gain in individuals who were started on an antipsychotic, as well as studies that focused on weight loss for patients who had previously gained weight. Interventions for both were found to be effective in the Alvarez-Jimenez meta-analysis. The Schizophrenia PORT (42) reviewed seven studies in which patients who were overweight were randomized to a weight-loss intervention or a control group. All of the studies found positive effects. Taken together, these studies provide strong evidence that clinicians should use these interventions when they are available.

Cognitive-behavioral approaches to managing weight seem particularly promising. For example, a study from the Diabetes Prevention Project (43) found that such an approach was more effective than metformin (described below) for weight loss and preventing diabetes. Weber and Wynne (44) modified this program for individuals with schizophrenia and found that it was effective. It was administered in 1-hour group sessions held over 16 weeks. Examples of the topics in these sessions include the following:

- Being active: A way of life
- Eating less fat
- Healthy eating
- Problem-solving
- Talk back to negative thoughts
- Managing stress
- Staying motivated.

*Adding metformin to the antipsychotic*: Metformin is an oral hypoglycemic that decreases hepatic glucose production as well as the absorption of glucose. It also increases insulin sensitivity. It is a useful drug for managing some type II diabetes as well as prediabetes. Randomized trials have found that doses of metformin between 750 and 2000 mg daily can be effective for reducing weight and improving lipids. Patients receiving metformin will often experience discomforting gastrointestinal side effects including flatulence, nausea, and diarrhea.

*Other approaches*: There are studies suggesting that adding aripiprazole to clozapine-treated patients can lead to weight loss (45). Other medications, including sibutramine and topirimate, have been tried with very limited success. None of these interventions—including metformin—is currently FDA-approved for metabolic risk.

## Tardive Dyskinesia

Tardive dyskinesias (TDs) are abnormal neurological side effects of antipsychotics that usually appear after years of treatment. However, some individuals will develop abnormal movements after just weeks or months of an antipsychotic. Common forms of TD include the following:

• Abnormal facial movements, including grimacing
• Abnormal movement of the jaw
• Abnormal mouth, lip, and tongue movements
• Choreoathetoid movements of the fingers and toes as well as the trunk.

Studies of patients on first-generation antipsychotics found that approximately 4% of patients each year developed TD over the first 5 years of chronic treatment (46). For patients over 55, the rate was substantially higher, approaching 25% during the first year. Patients treated with higher doses and patients who developed extrapyramidal side effects (EPS) were at a greater risk for developing TD. Treatment with second-generation antipsychotics appears to reduce the risk for TD, probably due to their lower risk of acute EPS (47, 48).

The great majority of TDs are mild or relatively mild. On the other hand, some TDs can be disabling. Patients may have abnormal gaits, odd truncal movements, and disfiguring facial grimacing. In most cases, the severity of TD develops and then stabilizes without progressing.

Common abnormal movements in tardive dyskinesia include the following:

• Buccolinguomasticatory movements
  • Sucking, smacking of *lips*
  • Choreoathetoid movements of the *tongue*
  • Lateral *jaw* movements
• Choreiform or athetoid movements of the *extremities* and/or *truncal areas*
• Any *combination* of these symptoms.

Clinicians who manage patients on antipsychotics should evaluate patients for abnormal movements on a regular basis. For patients who have been on antipsychotics for prolonged periods, an annual examination will probably suffice. More frequent examinations—every 4 or 6 months—are probably appropriate for patients who are experiencing EPS or for those who have just started on an antipsychotic. Table 4.5 provides a recommended method for briefly examining patients for both acute and tardive movement disorders. As clinicians gain experience, the examination can be performed in 2 or 3 minutes.

| Table 4.5 Procedure for Brief Assessment of Movement Disorders |
| --- |
| **Akathisia** |
| Observe for restless movements |
| Inquire about difficulty sitting still, restless feelings, and pacing |
| **Rigidity and tremor** |
| Observe for spontaneous movements and tremor |
| Examine for cogwheeling |
| Observe arm swing and gait while patient is walking |
| **Tardive movements** |
| Observe abnormal face and extremity movements while patient is sitting still with feet flat and again while patient is distracted with alternating thumb and finger tapping |
| Observe truncal, pelvic, and arm/hand movements while patient is walking |

## Managing Tardive Dyskinesias

There are no definitive treatments for TD. If a patient develops a relatively mild TD that only their clinician can see, watching the movement and lowering the antipsychotic may be reasonable. Often TDs that are mild will not progress to more severe movement disorders. When easily observed or disfiguring abnormal movements are detected in patients who should continue to receive an antipsychotic, changing to an antipsychotic with a lower potential for causing EPS may be helpful. Although there are few studies evaluating the effectiveness of changing antipsychotics for TD, when taken together, they suggest that antipsychotics with low $D_2$ affinity and a low liability for causing EPS, such as clozapine and quetiapine, are associated with less TD. There are also some data indicating that these agents may be effective for reducing TD (49). The evidence is strongest for clozapine, which is probably the antipsychotic of choice for more serious TDs. Quetiapine may also be worth trying since it is easier to administer than clozapine. The time course of improvement is relatively slow, and substantial improvement may not appear for months or years. In some cases, reducing the dose of an antipsychotic may also be helpful for TD.

Other medications may be helpful in some circumstances. Tetrabenazine is a drug that depletes monoamine stores and is effective for Huntington's disease. Although it is effective for treating TD, it is expensive and it can lead to depression with suicidal behaviors (50). Benzodiazepines may be helpful in some patients, particularly those who have TD variant with akathisia. A Cochrane review (51) indicated that the results from controlled trials were mixed. Nevertheless, a trial of a low dose of a benzodiazepine such as clonazepam may be warranted when the abnormal movements of TD are uncomfortable or disfiguring.

A reasonable strategy is to consider changing to clozapine or quetiapine when TD is disturbing or disfiguring. If the movements are severe, tetrabenazine or a benzodiazepine should be considered. Although adding a high potency antipsychotic to the patient's medications or raising the dose of their antipsychotic may temporarily suppress severe abnormal movements, in the long run this will not lead to sustained improvement.

## Endocrine Disturbances

The most common endocrine effect of antipsychotics is prolactin elevation. Since prolactin secretion by the pituitary is inhibited by dopamine, potent dopamine blockers—particularly first generation antipsychotics FGAs, paliperidone, and risperidone—increase circulating prolactin levels. Other antipsychotics, including most second generation antipsychotics, are associated with a much lower tendency to elevate prolactin. Prolactin elevations can lead to galactorrhea (abnormal lactation) and abnormal menstruation in women and sexual dysfunction and gynecomastia in men. Galactorrhea and gynecomastia can be disturbing and can lead to drug discontinuation. There are also suggestions that elevated prolactin levels may be associated with a small increase in the risk of breast cancer for patients on prolactin-elevating antipsychotics when compared with agents that do not increase prolactin (52). Finally, there are findings indicating that elevated prolactin levels may contribute to osteoporosis (53).

Prolactin elevations are also associated with sexual dysfunctions in both men and women (54). This is not surprising since prolactin elevations inhibit gonadotropin-releasing hormone and subsequently luteinizing and follicle-stimulating hormones. It is also important to point out that there are multiple possible causes of decreased libido as well as erectile and ejaculatory dysfunction.

When patients complain of symptoms that may be related to prolactin elevation, a prolactin level is easy to obtain. Normal prolactin levels are 5–20 ng/ml. Since a number of factors such as stress and exercise can elevate prolactin, levels under 40 should probably be repeated. Very high levels—such as above 200 ng/ml—should be evaluated by an endocrinologist since this may represent an adenoma. If the prolactin is elevated, patients can be changed to an antipsychotic with a decreased liability for raising prolactin. Among the SGAs, risperidone and paliperidone are the most likely to elevate prolactin. Clozapine, iloperidone, aripiprazole, and quetiapine are least likely to elevate prolactin.

If there are compelling reasons to continue a patient on the medication that is elevating prolactin, lowering the antipsychotic dose may be helpful. Alternatively, adding a low dose of aripiprazole—an antipsychotic that can lower prolactin—may be helpful (55).

## Cardiac Effects of Antipsychotics

Antipsychotic medications have the potential for prolonging the QT interval of the electrocardiogram, which, in turn, can result in torsades de pointes,

| Table 4.6 QTc Prolongation on 5 Antipsychotics in Milliseconds | |
|---|---|
| Thioridazine | 30.1 msec |
| Ziprasidone | 15.9 |
| Haloperidol | 7.1 |
| Quetiapine | 5.7 |
| Olanzapine | 1.7 |

a potentially fatal ventricular tachycardia. (Publications usually refer to the QTc, which corrects the interval for the heart rate.) This effect of an anti-psychotic is probably a major factor contributing to the association of some antipsychotics—particularly thioridazine—with sudden cardiac death. A QTc of about 400 ms is considered normal, while a level over 500 increases the likely of an arrhythmia. Antipsychotic medications differ in their tendency to prolong the QTc. One study (56) randomly assigned patients to a number of commonly prescribed antipsychotics and evaluated the QTc at the maximum plasma concentration. As noted in Table 4.6, thioridazine was associated with the greatest prolongation of the QTc.

These observations of QTc prolongation explain why thioridazine is now currently a second-line antipsychotic that should only be prescribed when others are ineffective. Droperidol has a similar restriction.

This information about QTc suggests the following management strategy. Although obtaining an EKG before starting an antipsychotic is preferred, it is not necessary when treating most healthy patients who do not have a cardiac history. Thioridazine and mesoridazine are associated with a cardiac risk and should probably not be selected for patients with or without a cardiac history, except when no other antipsychotic is effective or tolerated. If a patient in any age group has a history of cardiac risk factors such as diagnosed heart disease, a history of syncope, a family history of sudden death, or congenital prolonged QT syndrome, then an EKG should be obtained and reviewed. Since clozapine is associated with some QT prolongation as well as other cardiac risk factors including myocarditis, an EKG should be obtained before prescribing the first clozapine dose. Clinicians should also be concerned about QTc prolongation for patients who have a history of cardiac disease who are being treated with ziprasidone or iloperidone since they can prolong the QTc. It is also important for clinicians to be aware when patients are receiving medications other than the antipsychotic that also prolong the QTc or that inhibit the metabolism of the antipsychotic. For these patients, monitoring the QTc before and after starting the antipsychotic may identify patients at a heightened risk for arrhythmias.

## Non-pharmacological Interventions to Improve Functioning

Nearly every person with schizophrenia who is stable on an antipsychotic and who has impairments in their community functioning will benefit from some type of psychosocial treatment. The selection of the intervention should be based on the types of impairments of an individual patient. Box 4.1 lists the treatments that the Schizophrenia PORT has identified as meeting their criteria for having a sufficient evidence base. Cognitive behavioral therapy (CBT) is an approach to treating psychotic symptoms that persist when patients are treated with an antipsychotic. This approach is discussed in Chapter 6. Assertive community treatment, a strategy for patients who are high utilizers of mental health services due to frequent hospitalizations or homelessness, is also discussed in Chapter 6. Psychosocial interventions for weight management are discussed under metabolic side effects in this chapter. Psychosocial interventions for alcohol and substance use disorders are discussed in Chapter 6. Token economy interventions are effective in long-term inpatient facilities and are not discussed in this volume.

## Supported Employment

Supported employment is an approach to assisting patients to both find competitive employment and to maintain jobs once they are employed. It differs from traditional vocational rehabilitation in a number of respects. Rather than a period of assessment and job training, patients in supported employment begin a job search almost immediately. Rather than focusing on protected job settings such as sheltered workshops, supported employment focuses on competitive employment in the community. It also emphasizes finding a job setting where the patient is most likely to succeed. The specialist also provides support during the process of applying for a job and being interviewed. Once the patient has obtained a job, the employment specialist provides ongoing supports. If the patient agrees that his or her status can be disclosed, the specialist may also work with the patient's employer to address issues that arise in the workplace.

Controlled studies provide strong support for the effectiveness of supported employment in helping patients obtain competitive jobs, earn higher wages, and work more hours (57). There are also effects of obtaining a job that are difficult to quantify. Patients who work—even at part-time jobs—are better integrated into their communities and have enhanced self-esteem.

Clinicians should consider asking unemployed patients if they wish to secure a job. If supported employment is available, it is likely the preferred vocational intervention.

### Box 4.1 Evidence-Based Psychosocial Treatments from Schizophrenia PORT 2010

Assertive community treatment
Supported employment
Skills training
Cognitive behavioral therapy
Token economy interventions
Family-based services
Psychosocial interventions for alcohol and substance use disorders
Psychosocial interventions for weight management

### Skills Training

Skills training—also called social skills training, or SST—strategies use behavioral approaches to address interpersonal skills that are frequently impaired in schizophrenia. Elements of a widely disseminated SST program include basic perceptual skills, conversational skills, communal living, friendship and dating, communicating with health providers, vocational skills, and addressing drugs and alcohol. Patients are usually treated in a group format according to a written manual. Role playing and rehearsals are components of the training sessions. In addition, patients are commonly given homework assignments.

There is convincing evidence that patients who receive SST are able to learn important social and living skills. Obtaining these skills is associated with improvements in community functioning (42). SST is often provided in a group setting and administered by specially trained staff without doctoral degrees. Referral to SST should be considered for any patient with schizophrenia who has limitations in his or her social or life skills. This should include individuals with a range of functioning, from those who are attempting to adjust in school or the workplace to those who have the goal of living independently.

### Family-Based Interventions

A number of family-based interventions are recommended for patients who have substantial contact with family members and significant others. These interventions vary, with some focusing on providing education for patients and family members and others having broader goals including addressing crises, providing support, and other issues. The review by the Schizophrenia PORT notes that the results are clearest for interventions that are 6 months or longer. In these studies, family interventions were effective for reducing relapses and re-hospitalizations. There is also evidence that briefer interventions are also effective. Among the benefits for patients who receive family treatments are better treatment adherence and symptom reduction. Participating families also showed a reduced family burden.

## Key Points for the Stable Phase and Recovery

- The goals of treatment during the stable phase are to prevent a relapse in psychotic symptoms, to manage symptoms that persist, and to assist patients in meeting their own goals for recovery.
- Managing non-adherence with medications is the most effective means for preventing relapse.
- Long-acting injectable antipsychotics should be considered for patients with a history of non-adherence.
- Managing negative symptoms, cognitive impairments, and depression can improve the functioning of stable patients.
- During the stable phase, patients should be monitored on a regular basis for metabolic risk and neurological symptoms.
- Nearly every patient with stable schizophrenia will benefit from the addition of a recovery-oriented psychosocial treatment.

# References

1. Bratti IM, Kane JM, Marder SR. Chronic restlessness with antipsychotics. *Am J Psychiat.* 2007;164(11):1648–1654.

2. Barber ME. Recovery as the new medical model for psychiatry. *Psychiatr Serv.* 2012;63(3):277–279.

3. Leucht S, et al. Maintenance treatment with antipsychotic drugs for schizophrenia. *Cochrane Database Syst Rev.* 2012;5:CD008016.

4. Davis JM, Andriukaitis S. The natural course of schizophrenia and effective maintenance drug treatment. *J Clin Psychopharmacol.* 1986;6(1 Suppl):2S–10S.

5. Hogarty GE, et al. Drug discontinuation among long term, successfully maintained schizophrenic outpatients. *Dis Nerv Syst.* 1976;37(9):494–500.

6. Johnson DA, et al. The discontinuance of maintenance neuroleptic therapy in chronic schizophrenic patients: drug and social consequences. *Acta Psychiatr Scand.* 1983;67(5):339–352.

7. Weiden PJ. Understanding and addressing adherence issues in schizophrenia: from theory to practice. *J Clin Psychiat.* 2007;68(suppl 14):14–19.

8. Valenstein M, et al. Antipsychotic adherence over time among patients receiving treatment for schizophrenia: a retrospective review. *J Clin Psychiat.* 2006;67(10):1542–1550.

9. Ascher-Svanum H, et al. Medication adherence and long-term functional outcomes in the treatment of schizophrenia in usual care. *J Clin Psychiat.* 2006;67(3):453–460.

10. Blackwell B. Treatment adherence. *Br J Psychiat.* 1976;129:513–531.

11. Tiihonen J, et al. A nationwide cohort study of oral and depot antipsychotics after first hospitalization for schizophrenia. *Am J Psychiat.* 2011;168(6):603–609.

12. Leucht C, et al. Oral versus depot antipsychotic drugs for schizophrenia--a critical systematic review and meta-analysis of randomised long-term trials. *Schizophr Res.* 2011;127(1–3):83–92.

13. Midha KK, et al. Impact of clinical pharmacokinetics on neuroleptic therapy in patients with schizophrenia. *J Psychiat Neurosci.* 1994;19(4):254–264.

14. Marder SR, et al. Pharmacokinetics of long-acting injectable neuroleptic drugs: clinical implications. *Psychopharmacol (Berl).* 1989;98(4):433–439.

15. Herz M. Prodromal symptoms and prevention of relapse in schizophrenia. *J Clin Psychiat.* 1985;46(11 Pt 2):22–25.

16. Schooler NR, et al. Relapse and rehospitalization during maintenance treatment of schizophrenia. The effects of dose reduction and family treatment. *Arch Gen Psychiat.* 1997;54(5):453–463.

17. Herz MI, et al. Intermittent vs maintenance medication in schizophrenia. Two-year results. *Arch Gen Psychiat.* 1991;48(4):333–339.

18. Kirkpatrick B, et al. The NIMH-MATRICS consensus statement on negative symptoms. *Schizophr Bull.* 2006;32(2):214–219.

19. Rabinowitz J, et al. Association of prominent positive and prominent negative symptoms and functional health, well-being, healthcare-related quality of life and family burden: a CATIE analysis. *Schizophr Res.* 2013;150(2–3):339–342.

20. Faerden A, et al. Apathy in first episode psychosis patients: one year follow up. *Schizophr Res.* 2010;116(1):20–26.

21. Rabinowitz J, et al. Negative symptoms in schizophrenia: the remarkable impact of inclusion definitions in clinical trials and their consequences. *Schizophr Res.* 2013;150(2–3):334–338.

22. Gard DE, et al. Anhedonia in schizophrenia: distinctions between anticipatory and consummatory pleasure. *Schizophr Res.* 2007;93(1–3):253–260.

23. Grant PM, et al. Randomized trial to evaluate the efficacy of cognitive therapy for low-functioning patients with schizophrenia. *Arch Gen Psychiat.* 2012;69(2):121–127.

24. Green MF, et al. From perception to functional outcome in schizophrenia: modeling the role of ability and motivation. *Arch Gen Psychiat.* 2012;69(12):1216–1224.

25. Davis MC, Horan WP, Marder SR. Psychopharmacology of the negative symptoms: current status and prospects for progress. *Eur Neuropsychopharmacol.* 2013; e-pub.

26. Arango C, Garibaldi G, Marder SR. Pharmacological approaches to treating negative symptoms: a review of clinical trials. *Schizophr Res.* 2013 150(2-3): 346–352.

27. Elis O, Caponigro JM, Kring AM. Psychosocial treatments for negative symptoms in schizophrenia: current practices and future directions. *Clin Psychol Rev.* 2013;33(8):914–928.

28. Schaefer J, et al. The global cognitive impairment in schizophrenia: consistent over decades and around the world. *Schizophr Res.* 2013;150(1):42–50.

29. Kern RS, et al. The MCCB impairment profile for schizophrenia outpatients: results from the MATRICS psychometric and standardization study. *Schizophr Res.* 2011;126(1–3):124–131.

30. Green MF. What are the functional consequences of neurocognitive deficits in schizophrenia? *Am J Psychiat.* 1996;153(3):321–330.

31. Wykes T, et al. A meta-analysis of cognitive remediation for schizophrenia: methodology and effect sizes. *Am J Psychiat.* 2011;168(5):472–485.

32. Siris SG, et al. Depression in schizophrenia: recognition and management in the USA. *Schizophr Res.* 2001;47(2–3):185–197.

33. Whitehead C, et al. Antidepressants for the treatment of depression in people with schizophrenia: a systematic review. *Psychol Med.* 2003;33(4):589–599.

34. Marder SR, et al. Physical health monitoring of patients with schizophrenia. *Am J Psychiat.* 2004;161(8):1334–1349.

35. Newcomer JW. Metabolic syndrome and mental illness. *Am J Manag Care.* 2007;13(7 suppl):S170–S177.

36. Sikich L, et al. Double-blind comparison of first- and second-generation antipsychotics in early-onset schizophrenia and schizo-affective disorder: findings from the treatment of early-onset schizophrenia spectrum disorders (TEOSS) study. *Am J Psychiat.* 2008;165(11):1420–1431.

37. Practice guideline for the treatment of patients with schizophrenia. American Psychiatric Association. *Am J Psychiat.* 1997;154(4 suppl):1–63.

38. Meyer JM, Stahl SM. The metabolic syndrome and schizophrenia. *Acta Psychiat Scand.* 2009;119(1):4–14.

39. Stroup TS, et al. Effectiveness of olanzapine, quetiapine, risperidone, and ziprasidone in patients with chronic schizophrenia following discontinuation of a previous atypical antipsychotic. *Am J Psychiat.* 2006;163(4):611–622.

40. Stroup TS, et al. A randomized trial examining the effectiveness of switching from olanzapine, quetiapine, or risperidone to aripiprazole to reduce metabolic risk: comparison of antipsychotics for metabolic problems (CAMP). *Am J Psychiat.* 2011;168(9):947–956.

41. Alvarez-Jimenez M, et al. Non-pharmacological management of antipsychotic-induced weight gain: systematic review and meta-analysis of randomised controlled trials. *Br J Psychiat*. 2008;193(2):101–107.

42. Dixon LB, et al. The 2009 schizophrenia PORT psychosocial treatment recommendations and summary statements. *Schizophr Bull*. 2010;36(1):48–70.

43. Knowler WC, et al., Reduction in the incidence of type 2 diabetes with lifestyle intervention or metformin. *N Engl J Med*. 2002;346(6):393–403.

44. Weber M, Wyne K. A cognitive/behavioral group intervention for weight loss in patients treated with atypical antipsychotics. *Schizophr Res*. 2006;83(1):95–101.

45. Fleischhacker WW, et al. Effects of adjunctive treatment with aripiprazole on body weight and clinical efficacy in schizophrenia patients treated with clozapine: a randomized, double-blind, placebo-controlled trial. *Int J Neuropsychopharmacol*. 2010;13(8):1115–1125.

46. Kane JM. Tardive dyskinesia rates with atypical antipsychotics in adults: prevalence and incidence. *J Clin Psychiat*. 2004;65(suppl 9):16–20.

47. Woerner MG, et al. Incidence of tardive dyskinesia with risperidone or olanzapine in the elderly: results from a 2-year, prospective study in antipsychotic-naive patients. *Neuropsychopharmacol*. 2011;36(8):1738–1746.

48. Jeste DV. Tardive dyskinesia rates with atypical antipsychotics in older adults. *J Clin Psychiat*. 2004;65(suppl 9):21–24.

49. Remington G. Tardive dyskinesia: eliminated, forgotten, or overshadowed? *Curr Opin Psychiat*. 2007;20(2):131–137.

50. Aia PG, et al. Tardive dyskinesia. *Curr Treat Options Neurol*. 2011;13(3):231–241.

51. Bhoopathi PS, Soares-Weiser K. Benzodiazepines for neuroleptic-induced tardive dyskinesia. *Cochrane Database Syst Rev*. 2006;3:CD000205.

52. Azoulay L, et al. The use of atypical antipsychotics and the risk of breast cancer. *Breast Cancer Res Treat*. 2011;129(2):541–548.

53. Kishimoto T, et al. Osteoporosis and fracture risk in people with schizophrenia. *Curr Opin Psychiat*. 2012;25(5):415–429.

54. Rettenbacher MA, et al. Prolactin levels and sexual adverse effects in patients with schizophrenia during antipsychotic treatment. *J Clin Psychopharmacol*. 2010;30(6):711–715.

55. Chen CK, et al. Differential add-on effects of aripiprazole in resolving hyperprolactinemia induced by risperidone in comparison to benzamide antipsychotics. *Prog Neuropsychopharmacol Biol Psychiat*. 2010;34(8):1495–1499.

56. Harrigan EP, et al. A randomized evaluation of the effects of six antipsychotic agents on QTc, in the absence and presence of metabolic inhibition. *J Clin Psychopharmacol*. 2004;24(1):62–69.

57. Mueser KT, et al. Psychosocial treatments for schizophrenia. *Annu Rev Clin Psychol*. 2013;9:465–497.

# Chapter 5

# First Psychotic Episodes and Early Intervention

## Early Detection

Patients who have psychotic symptoms will often live with these symptoms for months, or even years, without treatment. This may occur for a number of reasons: individuals may not report their symptoms; the individual may not appreciate that symptoms such as suspiciousness are abnormal; or the person's treatment provider may not be experienced in managing psychosis. This delay in receiving treatment is important since there is a literature indicating that the duration of untreated psychosis (referred to as the DUP) is associated with a poorer outcome (1). Studies indicate that longer DUPs are associated with poorer social functioning (2) and a poorer response to treatment (3). One study from the United Kingdom found that a longer DUP was an independent predictor of outcome 10 years following the first admission (4). Taken together, these studies make a compelling argument for identifying individuals with a first episode and treating them as soon as possible.

The relationship between the DUP and clinical outcome has led to specialized programs that focus on the early detection and treatment of psychosis. These programs usually include public information campaigns that target young people and raise awareness of psychosis in schools and colleges. A study in Norway found that an early detection program was effective in improving clinical and functional outcomes (5).

## Management of Patients at Risk for Psychosis

The value of early detection has also led to strategies for identifying and treating individuals before the emergence of the first psychotic episode. The goal of the strategy is to prevent the emergence of a psychotic episode. Researchers in this area have struggled to find criteria that identify patients who are at a high risk for converting from a state where they are at risk to a psychotic state. The most successful criteria include psychotic symptoms that are below a threshold for actual psychosis, deterioration in social functioning, and a genetic risk for schizophrenia. Using these criteria, 30%–40% convert to psychosis over a 2–3-year period. About a third continue to be symptomatic, and an additional third recover (6).

Studies of intervening for the at-risk population have been somewhat mixed. A meta-analysis (7) found that antipsychotic medication reduced the risk of transition to psychosis by 45%. The number needed to treat (NNT) was seven, indicating that seven individuals would need to be treated to prevent one transition. The NNT for cognitive behavioral therapy was 13, indicating that it was less effective. However, these patients are sensitive to the side effects of antipsychotics. Studies also found that attrition rates were high among drug-treated patients. In one study that compared olanzapine or placebo in this population, there was some evidence that the antipsychotic reduced the prodromal positive symptoms. However, the olanzapine-treated patients had a mean weight gain of 8.8 kg (8). Given the limited benefits and strong adverse effects of antipsychotics, there is serious doubt as to whether individuals who are at risk for psychosis should be treated before they show clear symptoms of psychosis. Treating patients who are at risk with antipsychotics is currently considered off-label.

Pharmacological approaches other than antipsychotics have also been studied. Neuroprotection has been suggested as an approach for managing patients at risk for psychosis. This strategy is based on the research finding that the early years of schizophrenia are associated with losses in both gray and white matter. Protecting patients against these losses is a plausible approach to preventing or delaying the onset of schizophrenia symptoms. A recent study found that omega-3 fatty acids were effective in preventing the onset of psychosis in high-risk patients (9). This is a promising approach that hopefully can be replicated.

There is evidence that psychosocial approaches may be effective for patients at risk. A study from Germany (10) evaluated an intervention for at-risk patients that included cognitive behavioral therapy for psychosis, cognitive remediation, skills training, and multifamily psychoeducation. This experimental intervention was more effective than supportive counseling for delaying the onset of a first psychotic episode.

Taken together, these studies point to the importance of identifying individuals who are at risk for a psychotic break. However, the results of studies do not point to any particular strategy. Patrick McGorry and coworkers (11) have suggested a reasonable strategy for approaching patients who appear at risk. The strategy involves the initial use of safer treatments, such as a psychosocial treatment, followed by approaches with adverse effects, such as an antipsychotic, if second-line approaches are shown to be ineffective.

## Assessing a First Episode

An individual's first psychotic experience can be bewildering and frightening. It is not uncommon for both individuals with the symptoms and their families to delay seeking professional help, particularly when the symptoms are relatively mild or when the patient denies that something serious is happening. The early signs of the illness may be vague and may include social withdrawal, irritability, and deteriorating performance at work or school. In children and adolescents these symptoms may be falsely attributed to adjustment difficulties or reactions to stress.

Assessing patients with the first evidence of psychosis can also be challenging for mental health professionals. Management of the patient's symptoms may need to occur before a definitive diagnosis can be made. The assessment process should include the following:

- History of presenting symptoms (include informants such as family members when possible);
- History of substance use, head injury, medical illnesses, infectious diseases;
- Mental status examination;
- Physical examination with neurological examination;
- Laboratory: hematology, chemistry, and so on;
- Toxic screen if there is a suspicion of abuse.

The evaluator should ask directly about symptoms such as auditory hallucinations, suspicions, and unusual thoughts. Since these individuals may have never discussed their private experiences with a mental health professional, it may be useful to begin by asking about experiences that sound less unusual. For example, some people will have the sensation that something odd or ominous is occurring, which is discomforting. Others will feel that they are in danger without understanding the source of a threat. Some individuals may report that they are more sensitive to noise or more reluctant to go to crowded places. Early symptoms may include the experience that there is something odd about themselves. Some first-episode patients may respond negatively when asked about hearing voices, but they may have the feeling that they are hearing their own thoughts.

If it is possible and the person agrees, it is frequently helpful to involve other informants, particularly family members, in the evaluation. These individuals can provide valuable information about changes in the person's behavior. For example, it would be important to note if the person is misinterpreting what people are saying or if the individual is less interested in social activities or is becoming more isolated. It may also be helpful to use a long-term developmental perspective that focuses on a number of functions, including academic achievement, social skills, and recreational interests. In some cases, deterioration in these areas may have occurred well before the onset of psychotic symptoms.

Assessing substance use can also be challenging. Individuals may minimize or deny their use of drugs. This is particularly important for cannabis, which many adolescents and young adults view as a relatively safe drug. Moreover, individuals may fail to experience a direct relation between its use and symptom onset. However, there is evidence that the onset of psychosis with cannabis is associated with a cumulative toxic effect (12). As a result, individuals may not be aware of the relationship between use and the onset of psychosis.

## Diagnosis in a First Episode of Psychosis

The usual practice of beginning treatment after establishing a diagnosis is often impractical in first-episode patients. The differential diagnosis is likely to be relatively broad and may include substance/medication-induced psychotic disorder, schizoaffective disorder, bipolar illness, and other disorders. For many individuals, it may take months before a definitive diagnosis is possible. However, given the serious effects of prolonging the duration of untreated psychosis, as well as the dangerous behaviors that may occur in psychotic patients, it is almost always preferable to treat the psychotic symptoms before there is a firm diagnosis.

## Suicide and Self-Harm

First-episode patients have a relatively high risk for suicide. One study (13) found that 12% of first-episode patients showed suicidal behaviors. Risk factors for deliberate self-harm include alcohol and other substance use, greater insight, and depressed mood (14). It is important for clinicians who treat first-episode patients to discuss a patient's beliefs about his or her illness. During the early phases of treatment, expressions of hopelessness and despair should lead to careful monitoring of suicidal ideation. Management may include treatment with an antidepressant, assistance with efforts toward sobriety, and psychotherapeutic approaches to depression.

## Pharmacological Treatment for First Episodes

First-episode patients usually respond well to antipsychotic medication. Response rates tend to be higher than they are for multi-episode patients (15, 16). In addition, first-episode patients tend to respond to lower doses of antipsychotics, and they can be more sensitive to side effects (17). This sensitivity to side effects is a serious issue for individuals when they are first introduced to an antipsychotic. If they have discomforting side effects such as stiffness or akathisia, their attitude toward taking medication may be affected, for the first and future episodes. In addition, young people who are attending school or working may find even minimal amounts of sedation to be intolerable. Young men who experience sexual side effects or women who experience galactorrhea (or lactation not associated with breastfeeding after pregnancy) or irregular menses may also become non-adherent with their medications.

A number of studies compared antipsychotics in first-episode patients. A large European trial of 498 subjects (18) compared haloperidol, amisulpride, olanzapine, quetiapine, and ziprasidone over a period of 1 year. There were no differences in symptom reduction among the antipsychotics, although discontinue rates were higher for haloperidol. A comparison among antipsychotics in first-episode patients (19) found advantages in efficacy and reduced extrapyramidal side effects for olanzapine, amisulride, risperidone, and quetipine. However, there were greater increases in weight for olanzapine, risperidone, and clozapine.

Concerns about metabolic effects and weight gain should be an important concern in choosing an antipsychotic and a drug dose. Young people who

| Table 5.1 Weight Gain in 1 Year for First-Episode Patients (1) |
| --- |
| Olanzapine: 11–17 kg |
| Amisulpride: 10 kg |
| Clozapine: 10 kg |
| Quetiapine: 10 kg |
| Risperidone: 8 to 9 kg |
| Haloperidol: 4–11 kg |
| Chlorpromazine: 6 kg |
| Ziprasidone: 5 kg |
| Perphenazine: 1 kg |

gain weight, develop insulin resistance or diabetes, and have elevated lipids are at a substantially greater risk for premature death. In addition, weight gain in these individuals can have serious effects on their self-confidence and their social adjustment. Prior to treatment with an antipsychotic, first-episode patients are similar to healthy controls in their metabolic indices and weight. The cardiovascular risk increases after patients begin an antipsychotic (1). The changes occur rapidly. The systematic review by Foley and Morley found that the changes were evident at 1 month. In 6 to 12 months, weight increased by 10%–12%, along with substantial changes in LDL cholesterol and triglycerides. Table 5.1 lists the weight gain at 12 months for antipsychotics that were included in the review. The serious metabolic burden was also seen in a study with children and adolescents that compared molindone, risperidone, and olanzapine (20). The three antipsychotics were similar in their efficacy, but risperidone and olanzapine resulted in substantial weight gain. The weight gain and lipid elevations on olanzapine were severe and led the data and safety monitoring board to recommend that patients no longer be entered into the olanzapine arm of the study. This and other studies led the Schizophrenia Patient Outcomes Research Team (PORT) to recommend that olanzapine, along with clozapine, be considered as a second-line treatment for patients in their first episode (21).

The accumulation of research results from studies suggests a preferred approach for first-episode patients:

- Begin first-episode patients on lower doses;
- Do not choose clozapine or olanzapine as the initial antipsychotic due to weight gain;
- Warn patients about potential side effects and make adjustments to assure adherence;
- Inquire about side effects such as sexual dysfunction.

## Psychosocial Treatments for First Episodes

Nearly every patient who is experiencing a first episode will benefit from some type of non-pharmacological treatment. Educating the patient and usually the family about the illness will be important for every patient. Additional treatments such as interventions for weight management or substance use will depend on an individual's needs.

## Supported Employment and Supported Education

The Individual Placement and Support (IPS) model of supported employment (described in Chapter ) includes an individual specialist who works with patients to assess their individual goals, assist in placement at a work site, and provide follow-up supports after the individual finds a job. This model has been extended to include supported education for first-episode patients who are in a variety of educational settings (22). A study from Melbourne Australia (23) found that first-episode subjects assigned to these supports were more than 16 times as likely to be working or in an educational program when compared with usual treatment.

## Cognitive Behavior Therapy for Psychosis

Cognitive behavior therapy (CBT) for psychosis has been studied in patients at risk for psychosis as well as first-episode patients. One study (24) compared an intervention called Active Cognitive Therapy for Early Psychosis to a control condition. The cognitive intervention resulted in better early functional improvement. Although CBT has been shown to improve symptoms and improve quality of life, it has not been shown to prevent psychotic relapse (25). CBT has the advantage of providing tools for individuals to address their reality distortions as they emerge in the early stages of the illness. Conceivably these tools can help patients live with their symptoms even if medications are only partially effective.

## Family-Based Services

The great majority of first-episode patients are either residing with their families or are highly influenced by their families. There is very strong evidence indicating that interventions that educate family members about schizophrenia and help them to cope with the symptoms of the illness can improve patients' symptoms, increase patients' adherence with medications, and reduce the levels of family stress (26). Family to Family is a program developed by the National Alliance for the Mentally Ill. It is available without charge and is administered by family members.

## Alcohol and Substance Use

Substance use is among the common causes of relapse and rehospitalization in first-episode psychosis (27). It is also among the most common causes of self-harm (14). A review of substance use in first-episode patients (28) included individuals who were primarily users of alcohol or cannabis. It found that about half of patients became abstinent after an initial episode. It was unclear from the study if specific interventions were associated with improvement. The Schizophrenia PORT (26) recommends motivational and cognitive behavioral approaches to substance use in schizophrenia—without particular recommendations for first-episode patients. In addition, effective programs have usually integrated the management of the substance use disorder and the psychotic symptoms.

## Weight Management

As mentioned earlier, first-episode patients are particularly sensitive to the metabolic effects of antipsychotics. Moreover, weight gain can affect their long-term health as well as their self-image and their social adjustment. As noted in Chapter 4, there is substantial evidence supporting the effectiveness of a number of interventions for weight gain that is antipsychotic induced, including changing the antipsychotic medication, adding metformin or other agents, or behavioral-based interventions. Moreover, nearly all studies of multi-episode patients have found that behavioral interventions for weight loss are effective. There is some evidence that behavioral interventions for weight management can be effective for first-episode patients as well. A study from Spain (29) found that a lifestyle intervention was more effective than usual treatment for the 3 months during which subjects received the intervention. At 12 months, there were no differences between the groups, suggesting that the intervention should be sustained.

## Cognitive Remediation

The cognitive impairments in schizophrenia can be particularly damaging for first-episode patients who may be in school or in the workplace. As a result, there have been a number of studies of cognitive training in these patients, and the results have been encouraging (30). One study (31) found that cognitive remediation appeared to be more effective for improving work skills in recent-onset patients when compared with multi-episode patients.

## Family-Based Treatments

Individuals who are experiencing first episodes are much more likely to be in close contact with their families than are patients who have experienced multiple episodes. There is substantial evidence indicating that educating families about psychosis is effective in reducing the risk of a psychotic relapse and improving overall adjustment (32, 33). Multifamily psychoeducation groups that include both patients and their family members have been found to be effective and cost effective (34).

# Specialized Services for First-Episode Patients

Specialized teams have been developed for managing patients during their first episodes. In some cases, these teams have also focused on identifying patients at an early stage of the illness. Advantages of these teams include sustaining staff members who are knowledgeable about the challenges of treating first-episode patients and who understand the importance of family involvement. Experiences with these programs suggest that they are effective in preventing hospitalization (35, 36) and in improving outcomes. For example, a program from Melbourne, Australia, that included individual and family cognitive behavioral therapy was effective for preventing relapse in first-episode patients (37). The effectiveness of an intensive intervention for first-episode patients is currently being studied in a large randomized trial in the United States.

# Key Points for First Episodes and Early Intervention

- Decreasing the time between the first onset of psychosis and starting treatment leads to better outcomes.
- Individuals with first episodes of psychosis should be treated with an antipsychotic even before a definitive diagnosis is possible.
- First-episode patients often respond to lower doses of antipsychotics, and they tend to be more sensitive to side effects.
- Patients often fail to perceive the relationship between cannabis use and psychosis.
- Educating patients and family members about psychotic illness is an essential part of treatment.

## References

1. Foley DL, Morley KI. Systematic review of early cardiometabolic outcomes of the first treated episode of psychosis. *Arch Gen Psychiat*. 2011;68(6): 609–616.

2. Barnes TR, Leeson VC, Mutsatsa SH, Watt HC, Hutton SB, Joyce EM. Duration of untreated psychosis and social function: 1-year follow-up study of first-episode schizophrenia. *Brit J Psychiat*. 2008;193(3):203–209.

3. Fusar-Poli P, Meneghelli A, Valmaggia L, Allen P, Galvan F, McGuire P, et al. Duration of untreated prodromal symptoms and 12-month functional outcome of individuals at risk of psychosis. *Brit J Psychiat*. 2009;194(2):181–182.

4. White C, Stirling J, Hopkins R, Morris J, Montague L, Tantam D, et al. Predictors of 10-year outcome of first-episode psychosis. *Psychol Med*. 2009;39(9):1447–1456.

5. Larsen TK, Melle I, Auestad B, Haahr U, Joa I, Johannessen JO, et al. Early detection of psychosis: positive effects on 5-year outcome. *Psychol Med*. 2011;41(7):1461–1469.

6. Gee DG, Cannon TD. Prediction of conversion to psychosis: review and future directions. *Rev Bras Psiquiatr*. 2011;33 Suppl 2:s129–s142.

7. van der Gaag M, Smit F, Bechdolf A, French P, Linszen DH, Yung AR, et al. Preventing a first episode of psychosis: meta-analysis of randomized controlled prevention trials of 12 month and longer-term follow-ups. *Schizophr Res*. 2013;149(1–3):56–62.

8. McGlashan TH, Zipursky RB, Perkins D, Addington J, Miller T, Woods SW, et al. Randomized, double-blind trial of olanzapine versus placebo in patients prodromally symptomatic for psychosis. *Am J Psychiat*. 2006;163(5): 790–799.

9. Amminger GP, Schafer MR, Papageorgiou K, Klier CM, Cotton SM, Harrigan SM, et al. Long-chain omega-3 fatty acids for indicated prevention of psychotic disorders: a randomized, placebo-controlled trial. *Arch Gen Psychiat*. 2010;67(2):146–154.

10. Bechdolf A, Wagner M, Ruhrmann S, Harrigan S, Putzfeld V, Pukrop R, et al. Preventing progression to first-episode psychosis in early initial prodromal states. *Brit J Psychiat*. 2012;200(1):22–29.

11. McGorry PD, Nelson B, Amminger GP, Bechdolf A, Francey SM, Berger G, et al. Intervention in individuals at ultra-high risk for psychosis: a review and future directions. *J Clin Psychiat.* 2009;70(9):1206–1212.

12. Stefanis NC, Dragovic M, Power BD, Jablensky A, Castle D, Morgan VA. Age at initiation of cannabis use predicts age at onset of psychosis: the 7- to 8-year trend. *Schizophrenia Bull.* 2013;39(2):251–254.

13. Fedyszyn IE, Robinson J, Harris MG, Paxton SJ, Francey S, Edwards J. Suicidal behaviours during treatment for first-episode psychosis: towards a comprehensive approach to service-based prevention. *Early Interv Psychiat.* 2013; e-pub.

14. Challis S, Nielssen O, Harris A, Large M. Systematic meta-analysis of the risk factors for deliberate self-harm before and after treatment for first-episode psychosis. *Acta Psychiat Scand.* 2013;127(6):442–454.

15. Agid O, Arenovich T, Sajeev G, Zipursky RB, Kapur S, Foussias G, et al. An algorithm-based approach to first-episode schizophrenia: response rates over 3 prospective antipsychotic trials with a retrospective data analysis. *J Clin Psychiat.* 2011;72(11):1439–1444.

16. Robinson DG, Woerner MG, Delman HM, Kane JM. Pharmacological treatments for first-episode schizophrenia. *Schizophr Bull.* 2005;31(3):705–722.

17. Freudenreich O, McEvoy JP. Optimizing outcome with antipsychotic treatment in first-episode schizophrenia: balancing efficacy and side effects. *Clin Schizophr Relat Psychoses.* 2012;6(3):115–121.

18. Kahn RS, Fleischhacker WW, Boter H, Davidson M, Vergouwe Y, Keet IP, et al. Effectiveness of antipsychotic drugs in first-episode schizophrenia and schizophreniform disorder: an open randomised clinical trial. *Lancet.* 2008;371(9618):1085–1097.

19. Zhang JP, Gallego JA, Robinson DG, Malhotra AK, Kane JM, Correll CU. Efficacy and safety of individual second-generation vs. first-generation antipsychotics in first-episode psychosis: a systematic review and meta-analysis. *Int J Neuropsychopharmacol.* 2013;16(6):1205–1218.

20. Sikich L, Frazier JA, McClellan J, Findling RL, Vitiello B, Ritz L, et al. Double-blind comparison of first- and second-generation antipsychotics in early-onset schizophrenia and schizo-affective disorder: findings from the treatment of early-onset schizophrenia spectrum disorders (TEOSS) study. *Am J Psychiat.* 2008;165(11):1420–1431.

21. Buchanan RW, Kreyenbuhl J, Kelly DL, Noel JM, Boggs DL, Fischer BA, et al. The 2009 schizophrenia PORT psychopharmacological treatment recommendations and summary statements. *Schizophr Bull.* 2010;36(1):71–93.

22. Nuechterlein KH, Subotnik KL, Turner LR, Ventura J, Becker DR, Drake RE. Individual placement and support for individuals with recent-onset schizophrenia: integrating supported education and supported employment. *Psychiat Rehabil J.* 2008;31(4):340–349.

23. Baksheev GN, Allott K, Jackson HJ, McGorry PD, Killackey E. Predictors of vocational recovery among young people with first-episode psychosis: findings from a randomized controlled trial. *Psychiat Rehabil J.* 2012;35(6):421–427.

24. Jackson HJ, McGorry PD, Killackey E, Bendall S, Allott K, Dudgeon P, et al. Acute-phase and 1-year follow-up results of a randomized controlled trial of CBT versus Befriending for first-episode psychosis: the ACE project. *Psychol Med.* 2008;38(5):725–735.

25. Penn DL, Waldheter EJ, Perkins DO, Mueser KT, Lieberman JA. Psychosocial treatment for first-episode psychosis: a research update. *Am J Psychiat.* 2005;162(12):2220–2232.

26. Dixon LB, Dickerson F, Bellack AS, Bennett M, Dickinson D, Goldberg RW, et al. The 2009 schizophrenia PORT psychosocial treatment recommendations and summary statements. *Schizophr Bull.* 2010;36(1):48–70.

27. Addington DE, Patten SB, McKenzie E, Addington J. Relationship between relapse and hospitalization in first-episode psychosis. *Psychiatr Serv.* 2013;64(8):796–799.

28. Wisdom JP, Manuel JI, Drake RE. Substance use disorder among people with first-episode psychosis: a systematic review of course and treatment. *Psychiatr Serv.* 2011;62(9):1007–1012.

29. Alvarez-Jimenez M, Martinez-Garcia O, Perez-Iglesias R, Ramirez ML, Vazquez-Barquero JL, Crespo-Facorro B. Prevention of antipsychotic-induced weight gain with early behavioural intervention in first-episode psychosis: 2-year results of a randomized controlled trial. *Schizophr Res.* 2010;116(1):16–19.

30. Barlati S, De Peri L, Deste G, Fusar-Poli P, Vita A. Cognitive remediation in the early course of schizophrenia: a critical review. *Current Pharm Design.* 2012;18(4):534–541.

31. Bowie CR, Grossman M, Gupta M, Oyewumi LK, Harvey PD. Cognitive remediation in schizophrenia: efficacy and effectiveness in patients with early versus long-term course of illness. *Early Interv Psychiat.* 2013.

32. Onwumere J, Bebbington P, Kuipers E. Family interventions in early psychosis: specificity and effectiveness. *Epidemiol Psychiat Sci.* 2011;20(2):113–119.

33. Gleeson JF, Cotton SM, Alvarez-Jimenez M, Wade D, Gee D, Crisp K, et al. A randomized controlled trial of relapse prevention therapy for first-episode psychosis patients: outcome at 30-month follow-up. *Schizophr Bull.* 2013;39(2):436–448.

34. Breitborde NJ, Woods SW, Srihari VH. Multifamily psychoeducation for first-episode psychosis: a cost-effectiveness analysis. *Psychiatr Serv.* 2009;60(11):1477–1483.

35. Johannessen JO, Joa I, Auestad B, Haahr U, Larsen TK, Melle I, et al. First-episode psychosis patients recruited into treatment via early detection teams versus ordinary pathways: course and health service use during 5 years. *Early Interv Psychiat.* 2011;5(1):70–75.

36. Allott K, Alvarez-Jimenez M, Killackey EJ, Bendall S, McGorry PD, Jackson HJ. Patient predictors of symptom and functional outcome following cognitive behaviour therapy or befriending in first-episode psychosis. *Schizophr Res.* 2011;132(2–3):125–130.

37. Gleeson JF, Cotton SM, Alvarez-Jimenez M, Wade D, Gee D, Crisp K, et al. A randomized controlled trial of relapse prevention therapy for first-episode psychosis patients. *J Clin Psychiat.* 2009;70(4):477–486.

# Chapter 6

# Dual Diagnosis Patients

This chapter will address those patients with schizophrenia who also have a substance use disorder. The preferred substances of use, prevalence, risk factors, and treatment, as well as general principles regarding this dual diagnosis population, will be discussed.

Nearly half of those with schizophrenia will develop a comorbid substance abuse disorder at some point in their lives (1, 2); substances used are generally those that are most available and affordable (3). The rate of substance abuse is highest in those who are young, male, living in urban areas, homeless, incarcerated, or who began experiencing symptoms of schizophrenia at an early age (4, 5). Many cited reasons for drug abuse in this population are similar to those cited by the population in general: to experience euphoria, to socialize with a peer group, to decrease depression and low energy, and to obtain a general sense of relaxation. In some cases, hospitalized patients with schizophrenia and substance abuse disorders have also been found to have a lower level of negative symptoms (4, 6).

There are important consequences of substance abuse. Individuals who abuse substances are more likely to be treatment resistant and non-adherent to medications, and their rates of relapse are higher (4, 7). Substance abuse in combination with schizophrenia also confers a significant added burden of physical disease than that associated with either condition alone. Illnesses such as HIV, hepatitis, COPD, tuberculosis, and sexually transmitted diseases are all found at a much higher rate in dual diagnosis patients. Dual diagnosis patients have been found to have even further reduced levels of memory and attention than those with schizophrenia. The ability to maintain appropriate role functioning is increasingly diminished; this is further complicated by poor adherence to medications and psychiatric outpatient cares, contributing to higher rates of hospitalization. This itself is associated with more costly care, owing in part to additional diseases faced by this population (8–11).

In addition, patients with both schizophrenia and substance abuse disorders are more likely to be victimized, to be jailed, to become involved in violent situations, and to experience thoughts of suicide. Further, they are more likely to have difficulty maintaining employment, to become homeless, and to relapse if sobriety is initially gained (12, 13). These additional factors contribute to the grim reality that patients with both schizophrenia and substance use disorders are on average more likely to die approximately 12 years sooner than patients with schizophrenia alone; the risk of death by suicide in these patients is also increased (14).

The most commonly abused substances in this population, in order of use, are nicotine, cannabis, alcohol, and cocaine (1, 15, 16). Abuse of sedative drugs, methamphetamines, and opiates such as heroin exist but is less common. Each of these substances, as well as associated pharmacological treatment, will be discussed in turn.

## Nicotine

The prevalence of cigarette smoking in patients with schizophrenia is approximately 60%. The majority of these patients smoke more than one pack of cigarettes per day (17). This is in stark contrast to the general population, where the prevalence of cigarette smoking is estimated closer to 20%. Patients with schizophrenia have also been observed to take deeper and more frequent inhalations of cigarettes (18).

Those patients who are heavy tobacco smokers have been reported to experience more delusions and hallucinations as compared to those who do not smoke as heavily (18). Patients may also use nicotine as a way of lessening cognitive deficits and negative symptoms, such as lack of motivation and interest, that are associated with schizophrenia (4). Although cigarette smoking can improve cognition, the effects are transitory. As a result, there is no evidence that smoking can improve functioning.

Smoking is an important contributor to the high morbidity and mortality in individuals with schizophrenia. As compared to the general population, a patient with schizophrenia is twice as likely to die from cardiovascular disease and two to three times more likely to die from respiratory disease (10, 11).

### Management of Nicotine Use

Varenicline, bupropion, and various nicotine replacement systems (see Table 6.1) are available to patients with schizophrenia and substance use disorder (19). Given the significant burden of physical disease—including cardiovascular disease, cancer, and chronic lung disease—caused by smoking in patients with schizophrenia, it is important to consider these options as part of the overall treatment plan.

In the general population, varenicline can reduce craving and withdrawal symptoms associated with nicotine, and in patients with schizophrenia this drug has been shown to safely assist with quitting smoking at higher rates than those who do not use it (20). Of note, there is concern that varenicline carries with it the possibility of worsening psychosis (21). When prescribing this medication, it is good practice to discuss these and other side effects with the patient to ensure full understanding of this risk.

Bupropion also increases smoking abstinence rates in this population as compared to those who do not receive this medication, and without worsening psychosis (22). Since varenicline may be associated with a worsening of psychosis, bupropion is a reasonable first-choice agent.

Nicotine replacement using the transdermal nicotine patch also seems to be somewhat effective in this population, especially in those who are also taking second-generation antipsychotics (22), and the electronic cigarette may also be useful in decreasing the total number of cigarettes smoked per day. Other options include nicotine gum, lozenges, inhaler, and nasal spray.

Second-generation antipsychotics used to treat a patient's schizophrenia may also result in twice the smoking cessation rate as first-generation antipsychotics. Of note, many antipsychotics are metabolized more quickly in patients

## Table 6.1 Common Adult Dosing of Medications for Smoking Cessation

| Medication | Initial Dosing | Middle Phase Dosing | End Phase Dosing |
|---|---|---|---|
| **Varenicline** | | | |
| Initial | Days 1–3: 0.5 mg once daily | Days 4–7: 0.5 mg twice daily | |
| Maintenance | Day 8 and onward: 1 mg twice daily for 11 weeks | | |
| Varenicline note | Start 1 week before target quit date. Alternatively, patients may consider setting a quit date up to 35 days after initiation of varenicline | | |
| **Bupropion** | | | |
| Initial | 150 mg once daily for 3 days | | |
| Maintenance | Increase to 150 mg twice daily. | | |
| Bupropion note | Therapy should begin at least 1 week before target quit date. Target quit dates are generally in the second week of treatment. If patient successfully quits smoking after 7–12 weeks, may consider ongoing maintenance therapy based on individual patient risk:benefit. Efficacy of maintenance therapy (300 mg daily) has been demonstrated for up to 6 months. | | |
| **Transdermal nicotine patch** | | | |
| Patients who smoke >10 cigarettes/day (one-half pack) | Initial: highest dose of the nicotine patch (21 mg/day) for 6 weeks | Middle phase: followed by 14 mg/day for 2 weeks | End phase: finish with 7 mg/day for 2 weeks |
| Patients who weigh less than 45 kg or smoke ≤10 cigarettes per day | Initial: 14-mg/day for 6 weeks | | End phase: followed by 7 mg/day for 2 weeks |
| **Nicotine gum** | Recommended dose | | |
| Smokers who smoke 25 or more cigarettes per day | 4 mg | | |

(Continued)

**Table 6.1  (Continued)**

| Medication | Initial Dosing | Middle Phase Dosing | End Phase Dosing |
|---|---|---|---|
| Lighter smokers | 2 mg | | |
| Nicotine gum note | Smokers can chew one piece of gum every 1 to 2 hours over 6 weeks, with a gradual reduction over a second 6 weeks, for a total duration of 3 months. | | |
| **Nicotine lozenge** | | | |
| Smokers who smoke within 30 minutes of awakening | 4 mg | | |
| All other smokers | 2 mg | | |
| | One lozenge every 1 to 2 hours for 6 weeks, with a gradual reduction in the number of lozenges used per day over a second 6 weeks. The maximum dose is 5 lozenges every 6 hours or 20 lozenges per day. | | |
| **Nicotine inhaler** | 6 to 16 cartridges per day for the first 6 to 12 weeks, followed by gradual reduction of dose over the next 6 to 12 weeks. | | |
| **Nicotine nasal spray** | One or two sprays per hour are recommended for about 3 months. The maximum dose is 10 sprays per hour or 80 total sprays per day | | |

Source: Rind DM. Pharmacotherapy for smoking cessation in adults. In *UpToDate*, Basow DS (Ed.), Waltham, MA, 2013.

who smoke tobacco, making treatment potentially less effective. Patients should be asked about their smoking habits at every visit and medications should be adjusted as needed. The antipsychotics most susceptible to this phenomenon are clozapine, olanzapine, chlorpromazine, fluphenazine, and haloperidol (23, 24).

## Cannabis

It has been estimated that nearly 30% of patients with schizophrenia will use cannabis over their lifetime (16). Cannabis use also has been associated with an increased risk of developing schizophrenia (25) and at an earlier age (26).

There is a consistent association between cannabis usage, mostly during teen-age years or the early twenties, and the later development of schizophrenia (27). This risk is up to 200% higher among those who use marijuana heavily and who also start using at a younger age (28).

Cannabis is reported to be the drug most often associated with exacerba-tions of schizophrenia in some hospital emergency departments and acute psychotic episodes related to cannabis use yield poor overall treatment out-comes in this population (25, 28). Though perhaps obvious, given the serious implications for those abusing cannabis, clinicians would do well to remem-ber to regularly encourage psychotic patients to stop their use of cannabis.

### Management of Cannabis Abuse

While research regarding the treatment of cannabis use disorder in patients with schizophrenia remains limited, second-generation antipsychotics (and perhaps clozapine in particular) have been suggested to be most effective in reducing cannabis use in this particular population (4, 12).

## Alcohol

It has been estimated that approximately 20% of patients with schizophrenia will abuse alcohol over their lifetime (15). Patients with schizophrenia who also abuse alcohol have been shown to experience increased hallucinations, depression, and additional cognitive impairments, including difficulties with general problem-solving as well as difficulty following treatment recommendations (29, 30).

### Management of Alcohol Abuse

Medications are also available to address alcohol abuse in patients with schizo-phrenia, including naltrexone, acamprosate, and disulfiram, but the data are lim-ited. Naltrexone has been shown to reduce the overall number of days of heavy drinking and alcohol cravings in patients with schizophrenia and substance use disorder (31, 32). Disulfiram can also be successful in ultimately achieving remis-sion from alcohol abuse, despite many patients reporting ongoing use while taking this medication. Disulfiram, especially at higher doses, also carries with it the possibility of causing a worsened psychosis; again, clinicians should carefully discuss the possibility of this side effect with patients and monitor closely (33). Acamprosate can also increase overall length of abstinence from drinking, and may reduce psychological cravings for alcohol as well (34) (see Table 6.2).

## Cocaine

It has been estimated that approximately 15% of patients with schizophrenia will use cocaine over their lifetime (1). Those patients with schizophrenia who use cocaine show a lower level of overall functioning than those using other substances (35). Cocaine use in this population is also associated with wors-ened memory and increased depressive symptoms; the stimulant properties of cocaine can also worsen psychosis in patients with schizophrenia (36).

While limited evidence is available, second-generation antipsychotics used to treat the symptoms of schizophrenia also appear to be most effective in

| Table 6.2 Common Adult Dosing of Medications for Alcohol Abuse | | | |
|---|---|---|---|
| **Medication** | **Initial Dosing** | **Middle Phase Dosing** | **End Phase Dosing** |
| **Naltrexone** | Day 1: 25 mg | Maintenance: 50 mg /day | |
| **Disulfiram** | Initial: 500 mg once daily for 1–2 weeks | Maintenance: 250 mg once daily (range: 125–500 mg daily) | |
| Disulfiram note | Do not administer until the patient has abstained from ethanol for at least 12 hours. | Duration of therapy is to continue until the patient is fully recovered socially and a basis for permanent self-control has been established; maintenance therapy may be required for months or even years. | |
| **Acamprosate** | Oral: 666 mg 3 times/day | | |
| Acamprosate note | Treatment should be initiated as soon as possible following the period of alcohol withdrawal, when the patient has achieved abstinence and should be maintained if patient relapses. | | |

Source: Hermann R, Pharmacotherapy for alcohol use disorder. In *UpToDate*, Basow DS (Ed.), Waltham, MA, 2013.

reducing cravings and usage of cocaine (12). Treatment with the antidepressant desipramine in patients with comorbid cocaine dependence and schizophrenia may also facilitate less cocaine use overall (37) (see Table 6.3).

## Opioids

Though there has been limited study of treatment of opioid abuse in patients with schizophrenia, medications such as methadone, buprenorphine, and naltrexone have been used safely in patients with schizophrenia alone and could be considered in this population as well (9) (see Table 6.4).

### Treatment Strategies

As always, a thorough medical exam, including urine toxicology and physical exam, should be performed. It is also important to ask the patient for consent to contact anyone who might be able to provide additional details about his

## Table 6.3 Common Adult Dosing of Medications for Cocaine Abuse

| Medication | Initial Dosing | Middle Phase Dosing | End Phase Dosing |
|---|---|---|---|
| Clozapine | Phase 1: 12.5 mg once or twice daily | Phase 2: Increase, as tolerated, in increments of 25–50 mg daily to a target dose of 300–450 mg daily by the end of 2 weeks | Phase 3: May further titrate in increments not exceeding 100 mg and no more frequently than once or twice weekly |
| Clozapine note | May require doses as high as 600–900 mg daily (maximum dose: 900 mg daily) | | |
| Desipramine | Start at the lower range (25–50 mg/day) and increase based on tolerance and response | 100–200 mg/day, but doses up to 300 mg/day may be necessary in severely depressed patients | |

Source: Hermann R, Treatment of co-occurring schizophrenia and substance use disorder. In UpToDate, Basow DS (Ed.), Waltham, MA, 2013.

or her history; given the inherent difficulties in accurately recalling personal details of events that occurred while under the influence of substances, this type of collateral can provide very useful information not available elsewhere. While it may seem obvious, consideration must be given to keeping patients in treatment as long as possible. This increased time in treatment is associated directly with improvement, and this applies to nearly all drugs of abuse, including cannabis, alcohol, and cocaine (38).

## Psychosocial Interventions

Whenever possible, integrated care—treatment of both schizophrenia as well as substance use disorder by the same clinician or clinical team—should be offered. This type of treatment also places emphasis on patient and clinician engaging together in goal-setting within the setting of a nonjudgmental environment; in this way a therapeutic alliance can be developed via respect and empathy (9).

Individual interventions such as modified motivational enhancement therapy (MET) and modified cognitive behavioral therapy (CBT) have been used to treat patients with both substance use disorder and schizophrenia. Modified MET is an intervention that incorporates the principles of motivational interviewing to this dual diagnosis population, with the goals of exploring and facilitating engagement in treatment. For example, this has been shown to be effective in increasing abstinence and reducing number of drinking days in patients with schizophrenia who also had an alcohol use disorder (39, 40). CBT may also be an effective intervention in this population with

## Table 6.4 Common Adult Dosing of Medications for Opioid Abuse

| Medication | Initial Dosing | Middle Phase Dosing | End Phase Dosing |
|---|---|---|---|
| **Naltrexone** | Day 1: 25 mg | Maintenance: 50 mg / day | |
| **Methadone: short-term detoxification** | Initial: Titrate to ~40 mg/day in divided doses to achieve stabilization. May continue 40 mg dose for 2–3 days. | Maintenance: Titrate to a dosage which prevents/ attenuates euphoric effects of self-administered opioids, reduces drug craving, and withdrawal symptoms are prevented for 24 hours. | Withdrawal: Requires individualization. Decrease daily or every other day, keeping withdrawal symptoms tolerable; hospitalized patients may tolerate a 20% reduction/day; ambulatory patients may require a slower reduction. |
| **Buprenorphine** | Day 1: 8 mg | Day 2 and subsequent induction days: 16 mg; usual induction dosage range: 12–16 mg/day (induction usually accomplished over 3–4 days). | Maintenance: Target dose: 16 mg/day; in some patients 12 mg/day may be effective |
| Buprenorphine note | Treatment should begin at least 4 hours after last use of opioids, preferably when first signs of withdrawal appear. Titrating dose to clinical effectiveness should be done as rapidly as possible to prevent undue withdrawal symptoms and patient drop-out during the induction period. | | |

*Source:* Hermann R, Treatment of co-occurring schizophrenia and substance use disorder. In *UpToDate*, Basow DS (Ed.), Waltham, MA, 2013.

reducing substance use and decreasing troubling psychiatric symptoms, such as hallucinations and delusions.

Other interventions include peer support groups, which are similar to such existing programs as Alcoholic Anonymous but are modified to meet the cognitive and psychiatric limitations of patients with comorbid schizophrenia. Assertive community treatment (ACT) and case management programs are community-based interventions that can reduce homelessness in this vulnerable population while providing general life skills training (such as related to finances, navigation of transportation, personal care such as grooming and hygiene, etc.) to maximize chances of functioning in the community and minimizing substance use (10, 41, 42).

When various interventions of MET, CBT, skills training, and peer support groups have been combined, the outcome has been even greater. Decreased substance use, including fewer positive urine tests, reduced symptoms of schizophrenia, higher quality of life, and better adherence to treatment have all been observed with combination therapy (43, 18, 44, 45). Contingency management (CM) treatment, which involves offering patients tangible rewards to reinforce positive behaviors, results in more drug-free urine tests, longer participation in treatment, and total abstinence from drugs when added to the usual care of cannabis users. It has also been shown to generally reduce psychiatric symptoms, hospitalizations, and use of alcohol and stimulants in this dual diagnosis population as well (28, 46).

# References

1. Regier DA, Farmer ME, Rae DS, et al. Comorbidity of mental disorders with alcohol and other drug abuse. Results from the Epidemiologic Catchment Area (ECA) Study. *JAMA*. 1990;264:2511.

2. Kendler KS, Gallagher TJ, Abelson JM, Kessler RC. Lifetime prevalence, demographic risk factors, and diagnostic validity of nonaffective psychosis as assessed in a US community sample. The National Comorbidity Survey. *Arch Gen Psychiat*. 1996;53:1022.

3. Bradizza CM, Stasiewicz PR, Paas ND. Relapse to alcohol and drug use among individuals diagnosed with co-occurring mental health and substance use disorders: a review. *Clin Psychol Rev*. 2006;26:162.

4. Lybrand J, Caroff S. Management of schizophrenia with substance use disorders. *Psychiatr Clin North Am*. 2009;32:821.

5. Mueser KT, Essock SM, Drake RE, et al. Rural and urban differences in patients with a dual diagnosis. *Schizophr Res*. 2001;48:93.

6. Mueser KT, Drake RE, Wallach MA. Dual diagnosis: a review of etiological theories. *Addict Behav*. 1998;23:717.

7. Green AI, Tohen MF, Hamer RM, et al. First episode schizophrenia-related psychosis and substance use disorders: acute response to olanzapine and haloperidol. *Schizophr Res*. 2004;66:125.

8. Rosenberg SD, Goodman LA, Osher FC, et al. Prevalence of HIV, hepatitis B, and hepatitis C in people with severe mental illness. *Am J Public Health*. 2001;91:31.

9. Ziedonis DM, Smelson D, Rosenthal RN, et al. Improving the care of individuals with schizophrenia and substance use disorders: consensus recommendations. *J Psychiatr Pract*. 2005;11:315.

10. Himelhoch S, Lehman A, Kreyenbuhl J, et al. Prevalence of chronic obstructive pulmonary disease among those with serious mental illness. *Am J Psychiatry*. 2004;161:2317.

11. Dixon L, Postrado L, Delahanty J, et al. The association of medical comorbidity in schizophrenia with poor physical and mental health. *J Nerv Ment Dis*. 1999;187:496.

12. Brunette MF, Drake RE, Xie H, et al. Clozapine use and relapses of substance use disorder among patients with co-occurring schizophrenia and substance use disorders. *Schizophr Bull*. 2006;32:637.

13. Jones RM, Lichtenstein P, Grann M, et al. Alcohol use disorders in schizophrenia: a national cohort study of 12,653 patients. *J Clin Psychiat*. 2011;72:775.

14. Schmidt LM, Hesse M, Lykke J. The impact of substance use disorders on the course of schizophrenia--a 15-year follow-up study: dual diagnosis over 15 years. *Schizophr Res*. 2011;130:228.

15. Koskinen J, Löhönen J, Koponen H, et al. Prevalence of alcohol use disorders in schizophrenia: a systematic review and meta-analysis. *Acta Psychiatr Scand*. 2009;120:85.

16. Koskinen J, Löhönen J, Koponen H, et al. Rate of cannabis use disorders in clinical samples of patients with schizophrenia: a meta-analysis. *Schizophr Bull*. 2010;36:1115.

17. Chapman S, Ragg M, McGeechan K. Citation bias in reported smoking prevalence in people with schizophrenia. *Aust N Z J Psychiat*. 2009;43:277.

18. Ziedonis D, Williams JM, Smelson D. Serious mental illness and tobacco addiction: a model program to address this common but neglected issue. *Am J Med Sci*. 2003;326:223.

19. Tsoi DT, Porwal M, Webster AC. Interventions for smoking cessation and reduction in individuals with schizophrenia. *Cochrane Database Syst Rev*. 2013;2.

20. Williams JM, Anthenelli RM, Morris CD, et al. A randomized, double-blind, placebo-controlled study evaluating the safety and efficacy of varenicline for smoking cessation in patients with schizophrenia or schizoaffective disorder. *J Clin Psychiat*. 2012;73:654.

21. Cerimele JM, Durango A. Does varenicline worsen psychiatric symptoms in patients with schizophrenia or schizoaffective disorder? A review of published studies. *J Clin Psychiat*. 2012;73:e1039.

22. George TP, Vessicchio JC, Sacco KA, et al. A placebo-controlled trial of bupropion combined with nicotine patch for smoking cessation in schizophrenia. *Biol Psychiat*. 2008;63:1092.

23. Lohr JB, Flynn K. Smoking and schizophrenia. *Schizophr Res*. 1992;8:93.

24. Desai HD, Seabolt J, Jann MW. Smoking in patients receiving psychotropic medications: a pharmacokinetic perspective. *CNS Drugs*. 2001;15:469.

25. Dubertret C, Bidard I, Adès J, Gorwood P. Lifetime positive symptoms in patients with schizophrenia and cannabis abuse are partially explained by co-morbid addiction. *Schizophr Res*. 2006;86:284.

26. Arendt M, Rosenberg R, Foldager L, Perto G, Munk-Jorgensen P. Cannabis-induced psychosis and subsequent schizophrenia-spectrum disorders: follow-up study of 535 incident cases. *Br J Psychiat*. 2005;187:510–515.

27. Arseneault L, Cannon M, Witton J, Murray RM. Causal association between cannabis and psychosis: examination of the evidence. The British journal of psychiatry : the journal of mental science 2004;184:110–117.

28. Moore THM, Zammit S, Lingford-Hughes A, Barnes TRE, Jones PB, Burke M, Lewis G. Cannabis use and risk of psychotic or affective mental health outcomes: A systematic review. *Lancet*. 2007;370:319–328.

29. Pulver AE, Wolyniec PS, Wagner MG, et al. An epidemiologic investigation of alcohol-dependent schizophrenics. *Acta Psychiatr Scand*. 1989;79:603.

30. Manning V, Betteridge S, Wanigaratne S, et al. Cognitive impairment in dual diagnosis inpatients with schizophrenia and alcohol use disorder. *Schizophr Res*. 2009;114:98.

31. Petrakis IL, Poling J, Levinson C, et al. Naltrexone and disulfiram in patients with alcohol dependence and comorbid psychiatric disorders. *Biol Psychiat*. 2005;57:1128.

32. Petrakis IL, Nich C, Ralevski E. Psychotic spectrum disorders and alcohol abuse: a review of pharmacotherapeutic strategies and a report on the effectiveness of naltrexone and disulfiram. *Schizophr Bull*. 2006;32:644.

33. Mueser KT, Noordsy DL, Fox L, Wolfe R. Disulfiram treatment for alcoholism in severe mental illness. *Am J Addict*. 2003;12:242.

34. Ralevski E, O'Brien E, Jane JS, et al. Effects of acamprosate on cognition in a treatment study of patients with schizophrenia spectrum disorders and comorbid alcohol dependence. *J Nerv Ment Dis*. 2011;199:499.

35. Swartz MS, Wagner HR, Swanson JW, et al. Substance use and psychosocial functioning in schizophrenia among new enrollees in the NIMH CATIE study. *Psychiatr Serv*. 2006;57:1110.

36. Sevy S, Kay SR, Opler LA, van Praag HM. Significance of cocaine history in schizophrenia. *J Nerv Ment Dis*. 1990;178:642.

37. Ziedonis DM, Richardson, TE; Petrakis IL, Kosten T. Adjunctive desipramine in the treatment of cocaine abusing schizophrenics. *Psychopharmacol Bull*. 1992;28:3.

38. Horsfall J, Cleary M, Hunt GE, Walter G. Psychosocial treatments for people with co-occurring severe mental illnesses and substance use disorders (dual diagnosis): a review of empirical evidence. *Harv Rev Psychiat*. 2009;17:24.

39. Ziedonis DM, Stern R. Dual recovery therapy for schizophrenia and substance abuse. *Psychiatr Ann*. 2001;31:255.

40. Graeber DA, Moyers TB, Griffith G, et al. A pilot study comparing motivational interviewing and an educational intervention in patients with schizophrenia and alcohol use disorders. *Community Ment Health J*. 2003;39:189.

41. Brunette MF, Mueser KT. Psychosocial interventions for the long-term management of patients with severe mental illness and co-occurring substance use disorder. *J Clin Psychiat*. 2006;67(suppl 7):10.

42. Dixon LB, Dickerson F, Bellack AS, et al. The 2009 schizophrenia PORT psychosocial treatment recommendations and summary statements. *Schizophr Bull*. 2010;36:48.

43. Barrowclough C, Haddock G, Tarrier N, et al. Randomized controlled trial of motivational interviewing, cognitive behavior therapy, and family intervention for patients with comorbid schizophrenia and substance use disorders. *Am J Psychiat*. 2001;158:1706.

44. Shaner A, Eckman T, Roberts LJ, Fuller T. Feasibility of a skills training approach to reduce substance dependence among individuals with schizophrenia. *Psychiatr Serv*. 2003;54:1287.

45. Bellack AS, Bennett ME, Gearon JS, et al. A randomized clinical trial of a new behavioral treatment for drug abuse in people with severe and persistent mental illness. *Arch Gen Psychiat*. 2006;63:426.

46. McDonell MG, Srebnik D, Angelo F, et al. Randomized controlled trial of contingency management for stimulant use in community mental health patients with serious mental illness. *Am J Psychiat*. 2013;170:94.

# Chapter 7

# Special Populations

*Children and the Elderly*

## Children with Schizophrenia

The diagnostic criteria for childhood-onset schizophrenia is the same as is used for adult-onset schizophrenia, and the disease process is considered to be the same. However, those who develop schizophrenia as children will likely experience a more severe form of the disorder as they grow into adulthood. Of those with onset of psychotic symptoms prior to age 13, over half were found to have language, motor, and social abnormalities, and approximately one-third had academic difficulties prior to diagnosis (1–4). These children who are diagnosed with schizophrenia are approximately twice as likely to have a parent with a psychotic-spectrum disorder than those who develop schizophrenia as adults (5). Also, 25% of those determined to have childhood schizophrenia were at one point given an autism-spectrum diagnosis (6).

The prodromal phase of childhood schizophrenia is marked by diminished school performance, poor impulse control, increased aggression and hostility, and bizarre behaviors, including altered eating and hygiene habits (7, 8). Auditory hallucinations have been the most reported positive symptom, and these are simple rather than conversational or commenting voices. Delusions are the next most commonly reported symptom and often incorporate childhood material (i.e., frightening cartoon or movie characters). The majority of patients exhibit negative symptoms with flat affect, avolition, and poverty of speech most observed (9–12).

Childhood and adolescent-onset disease clinically present very similarly, but the timing of onset can vary markedly; childhood disease is characterized as being more insidious rather than acute, perhaps contributing to underdiagnosis and delayed treatment (13).

### Differential Diagnosis

Psychotic symptoms have been reported by nearly 10% of children without mental illness. These are most often experienced as hallucinations and delusions and occur without the concurrent bizarre behavior or deterioration in functioning seen in those with mental illness (14).

A number of other primary childhood psychiatric disorders can share symptoms of schizophrenia. The most common differential diagnoses include the childhood anxiety disorders, including obsessive-compulsive and post-traumatic stress disorders, and mood disorders of depression and bipolar disorder, as well as pervasive developmental disorders.

### Obsessive-Compulsive Disorder

Younger children with obsessive-compulsive disorder (OCD) may describe their intrusive thoughts as internal or external "voices," and this report may lead to a misinterpretation as hallucinations. In these cases, diagnostic confusion may occur between a severe OCD with lack of insight and a schizophrenic spectrum disorder with a psychotic delusion. In fact, those children with severe OCD may benefit from antipsychotic medication for their extreme anxiety (15).

### Post-Traumatic Stress Disorder

Children with post-traumatic stress disorder (PTSD) can have intrusive thoughts, vivid recollections, and derealization or depersonalization, symptoms uncommon to patients with schizophrenia. While hallucinations may be reported by children with PTSD, the content of these is usually related to some aspect of an antecedent trauma. Increased alertness and startle reactions may be prominent, which are also unusual in schizophrenia. Impaired attention and memory and suspiciousness, as well as irritability or aggression, impulsivity, and temper tantrums may be present; while these symptoms can overlap with schizophrenia, in PTSD many of the symptoms are related to an identified trigger or traumatic event (16, 17).

### Depression

While children with depression can experience associated psychotic features of hallucinations and delusions, unlike those with schizophrenia, children with psychotic depression usually do not demonstrate significantly disorganized speech or behaviors. Auditory hallucinations are usually reported to be mood congruent and, importantly, psychotic symptoms are noted only while mood is depressed (18–20).

### Bipolar Disorder

Children with bipolar disorder are more likely to have attention deficit hyperactivity disorder (ADHD) symptoms prior to diagnosis. A family history of bipolar disorder is also helpful in pointing toward an affective disorder. In comparison, children with schizophrenia have more frequent premorbid personality abnormalities and developmental disabilities, as well as a more insidious onset of disease flatter affect, and more hallucinations and delusions than children with bipolar disorder (21–23).

### Personality Disorders

Schizoid personality traits in children include solitariness, unusual fantasies, excessive interest in unusual topics, increased sensitivity, and paranoid ideas and an unusual style of communication; continuation of schizoid personality disorder into adolescence and adult life is most often reported (24).

Schizotypal personality disorder is characterized by marked abnormalities in social and interpersonal behavior, cognitive and perceptual distortions, and transient psychotic-like symptoms. The most common clinical outcome for children with schizotypal personality traits is development of this disorder.

About one-fourth of these children may go on to develop schizophrenia or schizoaffective disorder (25, 26).

Borderline personality traits are the most frequently studied personality traits in children. During the natural course of the disease, brief episodes of psychotic behavior and thinking, associated with many affective features, are reported; however, the outcome is usually not toward a primary psychiatric disorder but is usually toward a fully formed personality disorder (27, 28).

## Treatment

Appropriate treatment involves both psychopharmacological as well as psychosocial interventions. Antipsychotic medications are effective for reducing psychotic symptoms and preventing recurrences. Five antipsychotics are currently approved by the FDA for use in children; aripiprazole, olanzapine, paliperidone, quetiapine, and risperidone. However, other first- and second-generation antipsychotics are also likely to be effective. The earlier and more effective the treatment, the better the long-term outcome related to symptom control, as well as connection with the mental health care system. Antipsychotics provide effective symptom control, and of these, risperidone and clozapine have been most widely studied. Clozapine is also effective—but it is not FDA approved in cases of treatment-refractory schizophrenia in children and adolescents (29, 30).

Similar—but often more severe—side effects are seen with children as with adults. The prevalence of extrapyramidal symptoms (EPS) is usually higher in children treated with first-generation antipsychotics. Tardive and withdrawal dyskinesias can occur after initiation of these antipsychotics and are potentially irreversible (31–33). Risk factors for the development of these include higher doses, longer duration, female sex, and prenatal complications. Risperidone has been shown to be associated with a higher frequency of EPS (34). Similar to adults, it is important to monitor liver dysfunction, weight gain, hyperprolactinemia, hyperglycemia, and hyperlipidemia in children. Children and adolescents have a higher liability to experience antipsychotic-induced hyperprolactinaemia, weight gain, and associated metabolic disturbances than adults. Olanzapine is associated with the highest weight gain and is considered as a second-line antipsychotic for children and adolescents (35).

Psychosocial treatments include strong familial support when available, education for caretakers, behavioral modifications, psychotherapy, academic modifications, and assistance and enhancement of social and cognitive skills.

## Elderly Patients with Schizophrenia

The number of patients aged 55 and older with schizophrenia is expected to increase substantially during the coming decades (36). This "late-life schizophrenia" population can be divided into two groups: those who are now middle-aged but were diagnosed in late adolescence or young adulthood, and those who were first diagnosed at age 45 or older. This latter category, also known as "late-onset" schizophrenia, is more common in women than men (37), and these patients are noted to have higher premorbid functioning, less negative symptoms, and higher neurocognitive abilities (38).

The clinical presentation of late-life schizophrenia is marked by positive symptoms that are actually less impairing and fewer in number than their younger counterparts (39–40). Unfortunately, however, negative symptoms are more likely to continue into late life (42). Neurocognitive functioning, a strong predictor of functional independence among older patients with schizophrenia, remains on par with the functioning seen among schizophrenia in younger patients (43, 44). While there are baseline mild to moderate neuropsychological deficits associated with schizophrenia in general, having late-life schizophrenia does not seem to be associated with increased risk of cognitive decline (44).

Older persons with schizophrenia are at increased risk of having comorbid medical illnesses; this vulnerable population, however, is somewhat neglected in the medical community. The most common cause of death in all patients is heart disease, but those with schizophrenia die on average 10 years earlier than the general population. Studies have shown that patients with schizophrenia who suffered a myocardial infarction were shown to have 60% less likelihood of receiving appropriate interventions, including cardiac catheterization, as compared to the elderly population without mental illness. The prevalence of serious lung diseases, including COPD, are also significantly increased in this elderly population, in some cases by as much as three to six times above the national norms (39, 45).

Other subsets of this population who remain vulnerable are older homeless patients with mental illness and women. Middle-aged and older women with schizophrenia are 25%–30% less likely to receive standard women's healthcare, including pelvic examinations, Pap smears, and mammograms. Of note, among the elderly mentally ill, those with depression are far more likely to receive primary care than patients with schizophrenia (46–48).

Another cause of death in elderly patients with schizophrenia is by suicide. While this population has not been well studied, risk factors in elderly patients with schizophrenia include past suicide attempts, low quality of life, depression, hopelessness, and poor adherence to medications (45). Clinicians should also continue to monitor for increasing despair or hopelessness as patients become more aware of their illness and its implications. Encouraging regularity with psychiatric follow-up, including medication adherence, and monitoring the existence of social support are important components of care in the elderly population.

## Antipsychotic Medications in Late-Life Schizophrenia

The use of first-generation antipsychotics in the elderly population has been associated with a greater than 20% increased incidence of tardive dyskinesia, a disorder resulting in involuntary, repetitive body movements. This incidence increases to over 50% in 3 years of cumulative treatment (36, 49).

This incidence of tardive dyskinesia in this population is significantly lowered with the administration of second-generation antipsychotic medications. Overall, however, there is little research specifically examining the effectiveness of available medicines on this specific population (39).

As previously discussed, this population is particularly at risk for comorbid medical problems, and it remains of concern that these medications cause additional alterations in cardiovascular and metabolic function, including impaired lipid profiles and diabetes (50, 51). These patients should be regularly monitored for these side effects and maintained on the lowest effective dose of medication. Of note, patients with late-onset schizophrenia (as compared to those with early-onset disorder) are seen to typically require lower daily doses of antipsychotic medications (52).

It is worth mentioning that a warning has been issued of a 1.6- to 1.7-fold increase in mortality rates and cerebrovascular events in older patients with dementia (who are often prescribed atypical antipsychotic medications to assist with associated behavioral disturbances). These studies were conducted with elderly patients with a wide variety of dementing disorders, many of whom were living in nursing homes and who had pre-existing vascular conditions such as hypertension and history of strokes (53).

# References

1. Hollis C. Child and adolescent (juvenile onset) schizophrenia: a case control study of premorbid developmental impairments. *Br J Psychiat.* 1995 Apr;166(4):489–495.

2. Kolvin I. Studies in childhood psychoses: I. Diagnostic criteria and classification. *Br J Psychiat.* 1971 Apr;118(545):381–384.

3. Nicolson R, Lenane M, Singaracharlu S, et al. Premorbid speech and language impairments in childhood-onset schizophrenia: association with risk factors. *Am J Psychiat.* 2000 May;157(5):794–800.

4. Watkins J, Asarnow R, Tanguay P. Symptom development in childhood onset schizophrenia. *J Child Psychol Psychiat.* 1988 Nov;29(6):865–878.

5. Nicolson R, Brookner FB, Lenane M, et al. Parental schizophrenia spectrum disorders in childhood-onset and adult-onset schizophrenia. *Am J Psychiat.* 2003 Mar;160(3):490–495.

6. Sporn AL, Addington AM, Gogtay N, et al. Pervasive developmental disorder and childhood-onset schizophrenia: comorbid disorder or a phenotypic variant of a very early onset illness? *Biol Psychiat.* 2004 May;55(10):989–994.

7. Asarnow JR, Ben-Meir S. Children with schizophrenia spectrum and depressive disorders: a comparative study of premorbid adjustment, onset pattern and severity of impairment. *J Child Psychol Psychiat.* 1988 Jul;29(4):477–488.

8. McClellan J, Breiger D, McCurry C, et al. Premorbid functioning in early-onset psychotic disorders. *J Am Acad Child Adolesc Psychiat.* 2003 Jun;42(6):666–672.

9. Russell AT, Bott L, Sammons C. The phenomenology of schizophrenia occurring in childhood. *J Am Acad Child Adolesc Psychiat.* 1989 May;28(3):399–407.

10. Green WH, Padron-Gayol M, Hardesty A, et al. Schizophrenia with childhood onset: a phenomenological study of 38 cases. *J Am Acad Child Adolesc Psychiat.* 1992 Sep;31(5):968–976.

11. McKenna K, Gordon CT, Lenane M, et al. Looking for childhood-onset schizophrenia: the first 71 cases screened. *J Am Acad Child Adolesc Psychiat.* 1994 Jun;33(5):636–644.

12. Spencer EK, Campbell M. Children with schizophrenia: diagnosis, phenomenology and pharmacotherapy. *Schizophr Bull.* 1994;20(4):713–725.

13. Russell AT. The clinical presentation of childhood onset schizophrenia. *Schizophr Bull.* 1994;20(4):631–646.

14. McGee R, Williams S, Poulton R. Hallucinations in nonpsychotic children. *J Am Acad Child Adolesc Psychiat.* 2000 Jan;39(1):12–13.

15. Masi G, Millepiedi S, Mucci M, et al. A naturalistic study of referred children and adolescents with obsessive-compulsive disorder. *J Am Acad Child Adolesc Psychiat.* 2005 Jul;44(7):673–681.

16. Donnelly CL. Pharmacologic treatment approaches for children and adolescents with posttraumatic stress disorder. *Child Adolesc Psychiatr Clin N Am.* 2003 Apr;12(2):251–269.

17. Famularo R, Fenton T, Kinscherff R, et al. Psychiatric comorbidity in childhood post-traumatic stress disorder. *Child Abuse Negl.* 1996 Oct;20(10): 953–961.

18. Calderoni D, Wudarsky M, Bhangoo R, et al. Differentiating childhood onset schizophrenia from psychotic mood disorders. *J Am Acad Child Adolesc Psychiat.* 2001 Oct;40(10):1190–1196.

19. Chambers WJ, Puig-Antich J, Tabrizi MA, et al. Psychotic symptoms in prepubertal major depressive disorder. *Arch Gen Psychiat.* 1982 Aug;39(8):921–927.

20. Ulloa RE, Birmaher B, Axelson D, et al. Psychosis in a pediatric mood and anxiety disorders clinic: phenomenology and clinical correlates. *J Am Acad Child Adolesc Psychiat.* 2000 Mar;39(3):337–345.

21. Werry JS, McClellan JM, Chard L. Early onset schizophrenia, bipolar and schizoaffective disorders: a clinical follow up study. *J Am Acad Child Adolesc Psychiatry.* 1991 May;30(3):457–465.

22. Faraone SV, Biederman J, Wozniak J, et al. Is comorbidity with ADHD a marker for juvenile-onset mania? *J Am Acad Child Adolesc Psychiat.* 1997 Aug;36(8):1046–1055.

23. Masi G, Perugi G, Toni C, et al. Attention deficit hyperactivity disorder: bipolar comorbidity in children and adolescents. *Bipolar Disord.* 2006;8(4):373–381.

24. Wolff S. Schizoid personality in childhood and adult life: III. The childhood picture. *Br J Psychiatry.* 1991 Nov;159:629–635.

25. Asarnow JR, Tompson MC, Goldstein MJ. Childhood-onset schizophrenia: a follow-up study. *Schizophr Bull.* 1994;20(4):599–617.

26. Asarnow JR. Childhood-onset schizotypal disorder: a follow-up study and comparison with childhood-onset schizophrenia. *J Child Adolesc Psychopharmacol.* 2005 Jun;15(3):395–402.

27. Ad-Dab'Bagh Y, Greenfield B. Multiple complex developmental disorder: the "multiple and complex" evolution of the "childhood borderline syndrome" construct. *J Am Acad Child Adolesc Psychiat.* 2001 Aug;40(8):954–964.

28. Lofgren DP, Bemporad J, King J, et al. A prospective follow-up study of so-called borderline children. *Am J Psychiat.* 1991 Nov;148(11):1541–1547.

29. Sikich L, Hamer RM, Bashford RA, et al. A pilot study of risperidone, olanzapine and haloperidol in psychotic youth: a double-blind, randomized, 8-week trial. *Neuropsychopharmacol.* 2004 Jan;29(1):133–145.

30. Kumra S, Frazier JA, Jacobsen LK, et al. Childhood onset schizophrenia: a double-blind clozapine-haloperidol comparison. *Arch Gen Psychiat.* 1996 Dec;53(12):1090–1097.

31. Kumra S, Jacobsen LK, Lenane M, et al. Case series: spectrum of neuroleptic-induced movement disorders and extrapyramidal side effects

in childhood-onset schizophrenia. *J Am Acad Child Adolesc Psychiat.* 1998 Feb;37(2):221–227.

32. Connor DF, Fletcher KE, Wood JS. Neuroleptic-related dyskinesias in children and adolescents. *J Clin Psychiat.* 2001 ec;62(12):967–974.

33. Campbell M, Armenteros JL, Malone RP, et al. Neuroleptic-related dyskinesias in autistic children: a prospective, longitudinal study. *J Am Acad Child Adolesc Psychiat.* 1997 Jun;36(6):835–843.

34. Mandoki MW. Risperidone treatment of children and adolescents: increased risk of extrapyramidal side effects? *J Child Adolesc Psychopharmacol.* 1995;5:49–67.

35. Kreyenbuhl J, Buchanan RW, Dickerson FB, et al. The Schizophrenia Patient Outcomes Research Team (PORT): updated treatment recommendations 2009. *Schizophr Bull.* 2010;36:94.

36. Jeste DV, Alexopoulos GS, Bartels SJ, et al. Consensus statement on the upcoming crisis in geriatric mental health: research agenda for the next two decades. *Arch Gen Psychiat.* 1999;56:848–853.

37. Palmer BW, Heaton SC, Jeste DV. Older patients with schizophrenia: challenges in the coming decades. *Psychiatr Serv.* 1999;50:1178–1183.

38. Palmer BW, McClure F, Jeste DV. Schizophrenia in late-life: findings challenge traditional concepts. *Harvard Rev Psychiat.* 2001;9:51–58.

39. Folsom DP, Lebowitz BD, Lindamer LA, et al. Schizophrenia in late life: emerging issues. *Dialogues Clin Neurosci.* 2006;8:45–52.

40. Harrison G, Hopper K, Craig T, et al. Recovery from psychotic illness: a 15- and 25-year international follow-up study. *Br J Psychiat.* 2001;178:506–517.

41. Palmer BW, Heaton RK, Gladsjo JA, et al. Heterogeneity in functional status among older outpatients with schizophrenia: employment history, living situation, and driving. *Schizophr Res.* 2002;55:205–215.

42. Heaton RK, Gladsjo JA, Palmer BW, et al. Stability and course of neuropsychological deficits in schizophrenia. *Arch Gen Psychiat.* 2001;58:24–32.

43. Eyler-Zorrilla LT, Heaton RK, McAdams LA, et al. Cross-sectional study of older outpatients with schizophrenia and healthy comparison subjects: no difference in age-related cognitive decline. *Am J Psychiat.* 2000;157:1324–1326.

44. Palmer BW, Dawes SE, Heaton RK. What do we know about neuropsychological aspects of schizophrenia? *Neuropsychol Rev.* 2009;19:365–384.

45. Auquier P, Lançon C, Rouillon F, et al. Mortality in schizophrenia. *Pharmacoepidemiol Drug Saf.* 2007;16:1308–1312.

46. Cuffel BJ, Jeste DV, Halpain M, et al. Treatment costs and use of community mental health services for schizophrenia by age cohorts. *Am J Psychiat.* 1996;153:870–876.

47. Wasylenki DA. The cost of schizophrenia. *Can J Psychiat.* 1994;39:65–69.

48. Bartels SJ, Clark RE, Peacock WJ, et al. Medicare and medicaid costs for schizophrenia patients by age cohort compared with costs for depression, dementia, and medical ill patients. *Am J Geriatr Psychiat.* 2003;11:648–657.

49. Sable JA, Jeste DV. Antipsychotic treatment for late-life schizophrenia. *Current Psychiat Rep.* 2002;4:299–306.

50. Jin H, Meyer JM, Jeste DV. Phenomenology of and risk factors for new-onset diabetes mellitus and diabetic ketoacidosis associated with atypical antipsychotics: an analysis of 45 published cases. *Ann Clin Psychiat.* 2002;14:59–64.

51. Jin H, Meyer J, Mudaliar S, et al. Use of clinical markers to identify metabolic syndrome in antipsychotic-treated patients. *J Clin Psychiat.* 2010;10:1273–1278.

52. Arunpongpaisal S, Ahmed I, Aqeel N, et al. Antipsychotic drug treatment for elderly people with late-onset schizophrenia. *Cochrane Database Syst Rev.* 2009;2.

53. Alexopoulos GS, Streim JE, Carpenter D. Expert consensus guidelines for using antipsychotic agents in older patients. *J Clin Psychiat.* 2004;65:5–99.

# Mental Health Resources

## Emergency and 24-Hour Resources

**National Suicide Prevention Lifeline**
1-800-273-TALK (8255)
1-800-SUICIDE (784-2433) http://www.suicidepreventionlifeline.org/
Counselors available 24 hours a day, seven days a week.
**Boys Town National Hotline**
1-800-448-3000
A 24-hour crisis, resource, and referral line accredited by the American Academy of Suicidology
**National Institute of Mental Health Information Resource Center**
(24-hour; includes national referrals)
1-888-826-9438
**SAMHSA's National Helpline** (also known as the Treatment Referral Routing Service)
1-800-662-HELP (4357)
A confidential, free, 24-hours-a-day, 365-days-a-year, information service, in English and Spanish, for individuals and family members facing substance abuse and mental health issues. This service provides referrals to local treatment facilities, support groups, and community-based organizations.

## Additional Hotline Information

- **Adolescent Crisis Intervention & Counseling Nineline**
  1-800-999-9999
- **Drug & Alcohol Treatment Hotline** 800-662-HELP (4357)
- **American Addiction Helpline**
  1-800-468-6933
- **Gay & Lesbian National Hotline**
  1-888-THE-GLNH (1-888-843-4564)
- **Gay & Lesbian Trevor Suicide Prevention Lifeline** 1-800-850-8078
- **Help Finding a Therapist**
  1-800-THERAPIST (1-800-843-7274)

- **National Alliance on Mental Illness (NAMI) Helpline**
  1-800-950-NAMI (6264)
- **National Runaway Safeline**
  800-621-4000
- **Sexual Assault Hotline**
  1-800-656-4673
- **Suicide Prevention Lifeline**
  1-800-273-TALK
- **Suicide & Crisis Hotline**
  1-800-999-9999
- **Teen Solutions Helpline**
  1-800-400-0900

## To Locate Mental Health Services

**Substance Abuse and Mental Health Services Administration (SAMHSA)**
Mental Health Treatment Facility Locator http://www.samhsa.gov/treatment/index.aspx
**Centers for Medicare and Medicaid Services (CMS)**
CMS is the federal agency responsible for administering Medicare, Medicaid, State Children's Health Insurance (SCHIP), and several other programs that help people pay for health care. http://www.cms.gov/
**US Department of Health and Human Services**
Health Resources and Services Administration
http://findahealthcenter.hrsa.gov/Search_HCC.aspx

## Resources for Children

**American Academy of Child & Adolescent Psychiatry**
http://www.aacap.org
**American Psychiatric Association**
http://www.psychiatry.org/mental-health/people/children
**National Institute of Mental Health**
http://www.nimh.nih.gov/health/publications/treatment-of-children-with-mental-illness-fact-sheet/index.shtml

## Additional Resources

**Substance Abuse**
**American Council on Alcoholism and Assisted Recovery**
800-527-5344
http://www.aca-usa.org/
**National Council on Alcoholism and Drugs**
Automated Referral Service
1-800-NCA-CALL (1-800-622-2255)
http://www.ncadd.org/
**Al-Anon / Alateen**
1-888-4AL-ANON (1-888-425-2666)
http://www.al-anon.alateen.org/
**SAMHSA Substance Abuse Treatment Facility Locator** http://findtreatment.samhsa.gov/

**Depression**
**Depression and Bipolar Support Alliance (DBSA)**
(800) 826-3632
http://www.dbsalliance.org/

**National Institute of Health Resources**

**National Institute of Mental Health (NIMH) Information Resource Center**

1-866-615-6464

www.nimh.nih.gov

**National Institute on Alcohol Abuse and Alcoholism (NIAAA)**

www.niaaa.nih.gov

**National Institute of Child Health and Human Development (NICHD)** www.nichd.nih.gov

**National Institute on Drug Abuse (NIDA)**

www.nida.nih.gov

**National Center for Complementary and Alternative Medicine (NCCAM)**

1-888-644-6226

http://nccam.nih.gov

## General Resources for Clinicians

**UpToDate®**

UpToDate® is an evidence-based, physician-authored clinical decision support resource.

http://www.uptodate.com/home

**Medscape Schizophrenia Resource Center**

http://www.medscape.com/resource/schizophrenia

**Medication Information**

http://www.drugs.com

Data on more than 24,000 prescription drugs, over-the-counter medicines, and natural products.

# Index